Medical Ethics

The Moral Responsibilities
of Physicians

Occupational
Ethics Series

Norman Bowie Business Ethics
Peter A. French Ethics in Government
Tom L. Beauchamp & Laurence B. McCullough Medical Ethics

Elizabeth Beardsley and John Atwell,
Series Editors

Library of Congress Cataloging in Publication Data

BEAUCHAMP, TOM L.
   Medical ethics.

   (Occupational ethics series)
   Includes bibliographical references and index.
   1. Medical ethics.   I. McCullough, Laurence B.
II. Title.   III. Series.
R724.B358 1984   174′.2   83-21260
ISBN   0-13-572652-2

Editorial/production supervision:
   Chrystena Chrzanowski
Manufacturing buyer: Harry P. Baisley

Printed in the United States of America

10   9   8   7   6   5   4   3   2   1

ISBN   0-13-572652-2

PRENTICE-HALL INTERNATIONAL, INC., *London*
PRENTICE-HALL OF AUSTRALIA PTY. LIMITED, *Sydney*
EDITORA PRENTICE-HALL DO BRASIL, LTDA., *Rio de Janeiro*
PRENTICE-HALL CANADA INC., *Toronto*
PRENTICE-HALL OF INDIA PRIVATE LIMITED, *New Delhi*
PRENTICE-HALL OF JAPAN, INC., *Tokyo*
PRENTICE-HALL OF SOUTHEAST ASIA PTE. LTD., *Singapore*
WHITEHALL BOOKS LIMITED, *Wellington, New Zealand*

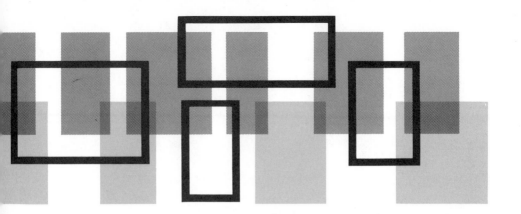

Medical Ethics
The Moral Responsibilities
of Physicians

TOM L. BEAUCHAMP
LAURENCE B. McCULLOUGH

Georgetown University

PRENTICE-HALL, INC., Englewood Cliffs, New Jersey   07632

for
Ruth and Linda

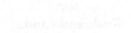

Contents

Prentice-Hall Series in Occupational Ethics

An increasing number of philosophers are coming to appreciate the value of making our discipline constructively available to those whose lives are chiefly focused on some form of practical activity. It is natural that philosophers specializing in ethics should be in the forefront of this movement toward "applied philosophy." In both writing and teaching many leading ethical theorists are currently dealing with concrete issues in individual and social life.

While this change has been taking place within the philosophic community, practitioners in various fields have (for several complex reasons) turned their attention to the ethical dimensions of their own activities. Whether they work in areas traditionally called "professions" or in other occupations, they wish to consider their job-related decisions in relation to ethical principles and social goals. They rightly recognize that many, if not most, ethical problems facing all of us arise in our occupational lives: we are often expected to conduct ourselves "at work" in ways which appear to conflict with the ethical principles believed valid in other social relationships; in our occupations themselves certain normally accepted practices sometimes seem to contradict each other; in short, ethical dilemmas of enormous proportion face the morally conscientious person. Whether philosophical ethics can help resolve these acute problems is an inescapable question.

A third recent development is the growing tendency of students to think of themselves as persons who do or will have certain occupational roles. This tendency is noticeable at several stages of life—in choosing an occupation, in preparing for one already chosen, and in pursuing one that has been entered some time ago.

The convergence of these three contemporary developments has created a need for appropriate teaching materials. The *Occupational Ethics* Series is designed to meet this need. Each volume has been written by a philosopher, with the advice or collaboration of a practitioner in a particular occupation. The volumes are suitable for liberal arts courses in ethics and for programs of preprofessional study, as well as for the general reader who seeks a better understanding of a world that most human beings inhabit, the world of work.

John E. Atwell and Elizabeth L. Beardsley, Editors

Preface

Moral problems that confront physicians range from the awesome to the routine. These problems are often complex and demanding, whether they occur in the dramatic setting of an intensive care unit or in the less hurried context of the family physician's office. This book is intended to provide a framework for addressing and, to the extent possible, resolving a wide spectrum of these problems. We emphasize that the title is *medical* ethics, while the subtitle refers to the moral responsibilities of *physicians*. Other books cover bioethics, nursing ethics, research ethics, health policy, and related subjects, but we make no attempt to treat this spectrum of subjects. Thus, we do not discuss such topics as the protection of human subjects of biomedical research or the moral responsibilities of biologists, nurses, and other health care professionals. Our focus is exclusively on clinical medicine and a clinically applicable account of the moral responsibilities of physicians.

Standards of moral responsibility and conflicts between moral principles are two persistent topics in this book. In pursuit of these themes, we base our inquiry on two potentially conflicting models of moral responsibility in medicine, each of which takes a different perspective on the *best interests* of the patient. One is the perspective of medicine, the other the perspective of the patient. The first five chapters address various themes of responsibility and conflict that derive from these models, while the sixth addresses the conflict that arises between the principle of promoting the patient's best interests and the principle of promoting the interests of third parties.

We develop all our analyses and arguments by reference to clinical cases. These cases are drawn from primary (office-based, out-patient care) as well as tertiary (hospital-based, in-patient) settings. Each case is based on actual events. However, the names of patients and physicians in the cases are fictional, with the exception of the two cases that introduce Chapters 1 and 4 and all cases drawn from the law (including the one that introduces Chapter 3). No violation of privacy or confidentiality occurs because names and other information are available in previously published material. We do, however, gratefully acknowledge receipt of new information directly from

Mr. Donald Cowart about his case, which appears at the beginning of Chapter 4. While no cases are hypothetical, the case that begins Chapter 2 is a considerably embellished and modified version of a case presented at a seminar held at the University of Michigan Medical School and arranged by Marc Basson. This source is not acknowledged in the text, but we do so here with appreciation.

In writing this book over the past few years we have benefited considerably from the comments and suggestions of colleagues and students who read the manuscript in its various stages. Several chapters were presented at seminars at the Kennedy Institute of Ethics, and others were presented in a number of seminars and colloquia at universities and medical schools. Many arguments were substantially changed as a result of the comments and responses of our critics on these occasions.

Physicians who read and improved the manuscript include Milton Corn, David Z. Meyerberg, Sanford Leiken, Tom Callahan, Barbara Jones, Arnold Siemsen, and Donald Seldin. Lawyers who saved us from numerous mistakes and oversights, while providing up-to-date legal information, were Alan Meisel, Judith Areen, and Nancy King. We also acknowledge the invaluable criticisms of Stephen Wear, Elizabeth Beardsley, John Atwell, H. Tristram Engelhardt, Jr., Ruth Faden, Warren Reich, Terry Pinkard, LeRoy Walters, and Robert Veatch.

As every teacher knows, students are often among the most perceptive critics of introductory textbooks. So it is with ours. Two graduate students, Ray Moseley and Donna Horak, and two medical students, David Doukas and James Nuzzo, were most helpful. They repeatedly forced us to make our arguments more available to students. No less important were the careful readings provided by Cathleen Kaveny, Linda Kern, and Timothy Hodges—three undergraduates with remarkably perceptive powers.

We also acknowledge with due appreciation the support provided to the Kennedy Institute by the Joseph P. Kennedy, Jr. Foundation. The Institute's library and information retrieval systems kept us in touch with the most important literature and repeatedly reduced the burdens of library research.

Finally, we make special mention of the extraordinary work of Edward J. Phillips, whose wizardry with word-processing equipment expedited the preparation of approximately eight very different drafts of this manuscript. His patience and perseverance cannot be too highly praised. Together with Chrys Chrzanowski and Mary Ellen Timbol, he also provided valuable editorial assistance that permitted the book to be cleansed of mistakes on a tight schedule. We are deeply grateful to all three of you.

T. L. B.
L. M.

Medical Ethics

The Moral Responsibilities of Physicians

Chapter 1

Moral Reasoning
in Medicine

An explosion of social, scientific, and technological developments has transformed medicine in the last half century, leaving the physician no longer predominantly a custodian and comforter. Powerful techniques of intervention have deepened and redefined our understanding of the moral responsibilities of physicians. Nonetheless, perennial moral problems have confronted physicians across the centuries. The following case is a dramatic example.

A CASE STUDY: NOTENCEPHALE

January 15, labor came on at one A.M. Having so often disappointed her friends, she waited until 4 A.M., when she requested that we might be summoned. Before the messenger had left the house, the head had passed the external organs. So little pain did she suffer in the descent of the head—the presenting part being very small—that she was deceived as to its proximity. Occurring in the night and residing a distance of a mile, half an hour elapsed before our arrival. We found the child born, completely enveloped in the membranes, with its lower extremities yet in the vagina. From the position, we concluded the birth had taken place with the face to the pubes. The membranes yet enveloping the head and body, were so entire and adhered so very close, that the least admission of air to the lungs was quite prevented. Two female friends were present, but they had offered no assistance. There was no pulsation in the funis umbilicalis. Discovering the monstrosity, we concluded not to attempt the inflation of the lungs; which would probably not have been successful for reasons to be mentioned when describing the brain. The mother felt the motion of its arms beneath the membrane for fifteen or twenty minutes after birth. . . .

The foetus, a female, very fat and perfectly formed, except in the parts to be described, measured thirteen inches in length, and weighed three pounds one ounce, and bore evident marks of having entered upon the eighth month of its existence. . . .

The vault or arch of the cranium fell directly backwards and downward from its brows; its cavity was very small, containing less than an ounce of the brain. . . .

1

The mass upon the back was at once recognised as the brain, covered with its appropriate membranes, through which the convolutions were distinctly seen, large, and imperfectly developed. . . .

The spinal column . . . was open throughout its whole length, the spinous processes being split in the middle (vertically) and turned so far to the right and left as to form a straight line with the posterior face of the bodies of the vertebrae, making a flat surface on which the base of the brain reposed. . . .

We see here the perfect integrity of the peripheral nerves, we see a tolerably well formed cerebrum, externally quite perfect, internally so soft that the minute subdivisions were not made out, as in a perfect brain. We learn, also, that there is no cerebellum, and no spinal cord. From the motions succeeding birth, may not the position be maintained, that there was a medulla oblongata, more or less perfectly developed, and if so, might not its seeing, hearing, smelling, and tasting, also have been moderately perfect? It would not have possessed the power of locomotion from there being no spinal cord; and although the organs of generation were perfect, yet, if the cerebellum holds that influence over their exercise which we believe it does, they could never have sustained their appropriate and important functions.

But we are going too far to suppose anything like the establishment of animal existence, where there is so signal a deficiency in the essential organs of the cerebral system, whose just adaptation to each other is so highly requisite to the continuance of the vegetative functions, the performance of muscular and sensitive motions and the more important manifestations of mental life.

From this and all similar cases, how irresistable the conclusion, that man, in his physical and moral nature, is admirably adapted to the sphere in which he exists, and the agents with which he is surrounded.[1]

This case of notencephale, and the attending physician's resolution of it, occurred in the early nineteenth century. It was published by Dr. Charles T. Hildreth (1798–1843) in Boston, Massachusetts, in 1834. The contemporary term for this infant's defect is "iniencephaly," a condition as untreatable today as it was a century and a half ago.

This infant's condition confronted Dr. Hildreth with a moral question: Ought he to have severed the membranes that covered the airways and that prevented the infant from attempting to breathe? The reasoning he presents in the case indicates that Dr. Hildreth was aware of this question. He first describes the patient's defects and makes clinical judgments about the diagnostic and prognostic implications of this infant's anatomical defect. Second, he uses these clinical judgments as a basis for *moral* judgments about whether medical intervention is in his patient's best interests. Let us reconstruct his moral argument in greater detail.

Because this infant suffered serious and extensive damage to her central nervous system, Dr. Hildreth did not attempt resuscitation. While he acknowledged that some parts of the infant's brain might have remained intact—e.g., those parts regulating the senses of hearing, smell, and

---

[1]Charles T. Hildreth, M.D., M.M.S.S., "Case of Notencephale, with Engravings" (Boston, 1834). Published privately for the author.

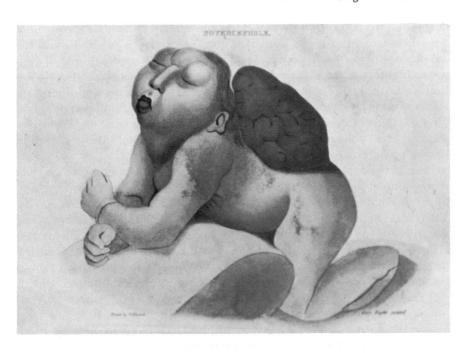

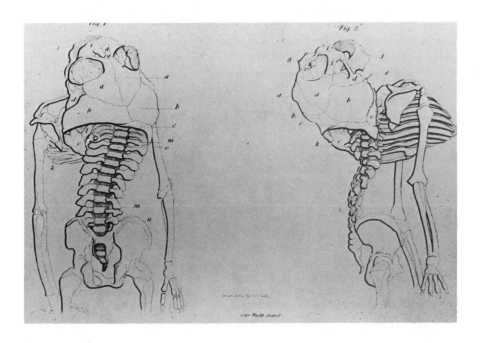

taste—he also noted that this infant would not be capable of locomotion. The damage to the spinal cord had created extensive paralysis, and the damage to higher brain centers would make even a minimal level of conscious life impossible. These observations led him to conclude that the infant would lack "the more important manifestations of mental life." This infant was barely capable of "animal existence" and had no hope of exhibiting the signs of distinctively human life. Dr. Hildreth reasoned that there was no moral obligation to attempt her resuscitation because it was not in her best interests to do so.

Even if the brain were intact and this infant were to enjoy more than mere "animal existence," there was then (and is now) no known medical intervention for successfully replacing the brain into the cranial cavity. Therefore, in addition to moral problems about whether the infant *should* live, there is the tragic problem that it was impossible to keep this patient alive for any significant period of time. For these reasons, too, Dr. Hildreth decided that resuscitation was not morally required and the infant should be allowed to die (or, as some physicians might hold, pronounced dead).

A century and a half after this case, physicians, families, and society continue to struggle with moral problems in the care of seriously ill infants. A case in the spring of 1982 known as "Infant Doe" received national attention and prompted strong conflicting responses. With the permission of an Indiana court, an infant with an esophageal-tracheal fistula[2] and trisomy 21,[3] a form of mental retardation (also known as Down's syndrome), was allowed to die at the request of the parents. In March 1983, in response to this and related cases, the United States Department of Health and Human Services issued an "Interim Final Rule" directing that, in all health care facilities receiving federal funds, the following public notice should be displayed in maternity wards, pediatric wards treating infants under one year of age, and neonatal intensive care units:[4]

DISCRIMINATORY FAILURE TO FEED AND CARE FOR HANDICAPPED INFANTS IN THIS FACILITIY IS PROHIBITED BY FEDERAL LAW.
Any person having knowledge that a handicapped infant is being discriminatorily denied food or customary medical care should immediately contact:
Handicapped Infant Hotline
U.S. Department of Health and Human Services
Washington, D.C. 20201
Phone 800-   (Available 24 hours a day)
or
Your State Child Protective Agency

[2]An esophageal-tracheal fistula is an anatomical defect involving an opening between the esophagus (passage to intestinal tract) and the trachea (the "windpipe," a passage to the lungs).

[3]Trisomy 21 involves extra genetic material in the 21st chromosome.

[4]"Nondiscrimination on the Basis of Handicap," *Federal Register* 48 (7 March 1983): 9630–32.

The text of the rule implicitly suggests that "customery medical care" in this context means medical treatment "essential to maintain life," or "to correct a life-threatening condition." This language seems broad enough to potentially include medical treatment for severe handicaps such as iniencephaly, anencephaly (absence of the vital parts of the brain), and massive cerebral hemorrhage.

Several organizations expressed opposition to this regulation, including the American Academy of Pediatrics and the American Medical Association.[5] However, other organizations endorsed the regulation, including the American Association of Retarded Citizens. Immediately after the rule was issued, a bill written along similar lines was introduced into the legislature of the state of Maryland. The legislation was designed to "prohibit doctors, nurses and midwives in Maryland from withholding food, water, or other 'things required for sustenance' from a newborn child in their care."[6] Similar legislation was introduced in both houses of Congress.

In sum, many now characterize the responsibilities of physicians in ways that depart from Dr. Hildreth's reflections. In light of the Interim Final Rule, for example, his appeal to the infant's lack of potential for "mental life" might not be accepted as legitimate. His reasoning suggests that this particular handicapping condition is a good and sufficient reason for withholding treatment because the patient cannot experience any benefit from its administration. As a consequence, Dr. Hildreth's understanding of his responsibility to his infant patient might be judged in violation of the law in the United States. This interpretation of law is built on civil rights statutes and, more generally, on the traditional legal theory that a failure to discharge a legal duty—either the parent's or the physician's—that results in another's death is first- or second-degree murder (depending on the degree of premeditation) or involuntary manslaughter because of gross carelessness. The law assumes that, following birth, a person exists with the full protection of legal rights. But are these legal principles adequate in these circumstances, and is the law authoritative for determining the moral responsibilities of physicians? Might not the more discretionary arguments of Dr. Hildreth be a sounder moral basis for reaching conclusions about moral responsibilities? Such questions about potential conflicts between the law and medical ethics will plague us throughout this volume. It must never be presumed that legal duties as such establish moral duties, or vice versa.

---

[5]Those opposed to the Interim Final Rule were successful in obtaining an injunction in federal court, which suspended the rule on narrow technical, procedural grounds. See *American Academy of Pediatrics, et al. v. Margaret M. Heckler*. Civil Action No. 83–0774, United States District Court for the District of Columbia (April 14, 1983). The secretary of the Department of Health and Human Services announced, however, that the government would appeal the injunction. The goverment reissued the rule in a new form in July 1983 [*Federal Register* (5 July 1983): 30846 ff].

[6]"Catholic Right-to-Life Groups Support Ban on Withholding Food for Newborn," *Washington Post*, 18 March 1983.

Dr. Hildreth's case report was published privately and so did not have the public impact of a court hearing, a federally promulgated regulation, or proposed legislation. Today there is greater public involvement in debates about medical ethics. Nonetheless, Dr. Hildreth's thinking about the Case of Notencephale anticipates our own. Much of the contemporary debate about the care of seriously ill infants centers on so-called quality-of-life considerations. Dr. Hildreth's concern with the possibilities of "mental life" foreshadows these considerations.

Many writers in medical ethics tend to believe that the rise of high medical technology—epitomized in the neonatal intensive care unit of a large, urban hospital—is a major and unique source of these moral problems. New medical technologies obviously extend the range of possible interventions beyond that of merely providing comfort—often all that could be provided in the past—and these technologies can also present a greater burden of pain and suffering, as well as psychological and financial costs, than the minimal technology of Dr. Hildreth's time. If the infant he attended were born today in a large urban hospital, there would be mechanical respirators to breathe for her. But should the physician direct that an infant with iniencephaly be put on a respirator? Would it be in the patient's best interests to do so? These questions are not new, for they directly parallel those facing Dr. Hildreth. Medical technologies have complicated ethical problems in medicine, but they are not always a *novel source* of those problems. Indeed, many of the moral questions physicians now encounter were encountered in some form centuries ago.

TAKING HISTORY SERIOUSLY

Problems about the moral responsibilities of physicians arise, we shall argue, as a result of competing perspectives on the patient's best interests—the perspective of medicine and the perspective of the patient. Many premises in our argument are developed from historical foundations because these two perspectives and the powerful models of moral responsibility in which they are expressed cannot be understood apart from their historical roots in medical, legal, and philosophical traditions. As we note in chapter six, the broad outlines of a physician's responsibilities in the Soviet Union are enormously different from those in Western democracies. Our histories and ancient traditions create this difference, even though we share similar modern medical technologies and medical problems in dealing with patients. We therefore take historical inquiry to be essential to contemporary medical ethics.

There has been a tendency in recent medical ethics either to ignore history altogether or to give it only a passing nod by acknowledging historical documents like the Hippocratic writings (fifth to fourth century, B.C.),[7] Percival's *Medical Ethics* (1803),[8] and the first *Code of Ethics* (1846–1847) of the American Medical Association.[9] One of the goals of this book is to redirect inquiry in medical ethics by taking its history seriously. To achieve this goal, we employ two primary forms of historical investigation.

First, the writings of the great figures in this history are a rich repository for ongoing work. While important writings are found in numerous ancient, medieval, and modern sources, in this book we concentrate on some of the major figures in two periods: ancient Greece and the Enlightenment to the present. We shall examine some of the Hippocratic writings, as well as those of major modern figures of the eighteenth and nineteenth centuries, including the British physicians John Gregory (1724–1773) and Thomas Percival (1740–1804); the American physicians Samuel Bard (1742–1821), Benjamin Rush (1745–1813), Worthington Hooker (1806–1867), Austin Flint, Sr. (1812–1886), and Richard C. Cabot (1868–1939); the Canadian physician Sir William Osler (1849–1919); and the German physician Johann Peter Frank (1745–1821). We will study, for example, the development of ideas about the physician's obligation to be truthful to the dying patient by examining some of the great traditional writings on this subject.

Another form of historical inquiry is to place traditional writings in their original contexts. For example, this method reveals that Dr. Hildreth's report was intended to be a contribution to the newly emerging science of birth defects, teratology. Further study would trace the sources for his understanding of the significance of "mental life" in the traditional, Aristotelian tripartite distinction among types or categories of living things: vegetative, animal, and human. This large task is beyond the scope of this book; we are examining medical ethics, not its history. Still, when it is important, we shall engage in limited inquiry of this sort. For example, this approach will prove invaluable in chapter two where we examine the historical roots of two models of moral responsibility in the histories of medical ethics, law, and philosophy.

The history of medical ethics has developed under a number of diverse influences and from a variety of sources. For example, the Hippocratic Oath was influenced by a religious sect known as Pythagoreanism. The views the Oath takes on abortion and on giving poisons to patients are par-

[7]W. H. S. Jones, trans., *Hippocrates* (Cambridge: Harvard University Press, The Loeb Classical Library, 1923).

[8]Thomas Percival, *Percival's Medical Ethics*, ed. Chauncey Leake (Huntington, N.Y.: Robert E. Krieger Publishing Co., 1975). Reprint of Percival's *Medical Ethics* (Manchester, England: S. Russell, 1803).

[9]American Medical Association, *Proceedings of the National Medical Convention, 1846–1847*, in *Ethics in Medicine*, ed. Stanley Reiser et al. (Cambridge: MIT Press, 1977), pp. 26–34.

ticular examples.[10] Later, especially in medieval Europe, medical ethics was deeply influenced by Christianity, which placed special emphasis on compassion for the ill.[11] During and following the Enlightenment, medical ethics drew on more secular sources, such as philosophy and law. Throughout this history two primary forms of writings and documents developed: The first is comprised of oaths and codes, an attempt to organize the moral responsibilities of physicians into a concise format. To this tradition belong the Hippocratic Oath and its descendents to the present day, as well as the various codes of ethics or "principles of ethics" of organized medicine—e.g., the first *Code of Ethics* of the American Medical Association and its successors. The second form of writing is a more literary, "learned" tradition, comprising discursive study of medical ethics through treatises and books. Our book follows this second tradition.

MEDICAL ETHICS
AND PHILOSOPHICAL ETHICS

While we take history seriously, we do not take history to be the exclusive source for moral reasoning in medicine. Instead, we situate our inquiry in a broader intellectual and social context, one in which medical ethics has developed and continues to develop in the context of morality generally, through philosophical reasoning and through the contributions of many disciplines. Because medical ethics is a continuing enterprise, it deserves as rigorous and systematic an analysis and development as possible. Let us begin by placing medical ethics within social institutions of morality familiar to us all.

The Nature, Origin, and Purposes
of Morality

The words "ethics" and "morality" in the English language are not confined either to abstract philosophical contexts or to narrow professional codes of conduct. Morality is concerned with right and wrong human conduct in general. The word "morality" denotes a social institution, composed of a set of rules that are generally acknowledged by its members. Like political constitutions and natural languages, morality exists before any individual is introduced to its relevant rules and regulations. It is transmitted from

---

[10]Ludwig Edelstein, *Ancient Medicine: Selected Papers of Ludwig Edelstein*, ed. Owsei Temkin and C. Lilian Temkin (Baltimore: The Johns Hopkins University Press, 1967), passim.

[11]Darrel Amundsen, "Medical Ethics, History of: Medieval Europe: Fourth to Sixteenth Century," in *Encyclopedia of Bioethics*, ed. Warren T. Reich (New York: The Free Press, 1978), p. 938.

generation to generation along with other societal customs and rules. We thus learn the rules of morality from many sources, including families, ethnic and racial groups, nations, organized religions, and legal structures.

Morality in the profession of medicine is similarly social. In the training of physicians, ethical precepts are often taught together with other rules of good medical practice and customs of the medical community. Indeed, it is sometimes difficult to distinguish a moral judgment in medicine from a judgment of due care or appropriate medical practice. For example, medical students learn a moral point of view when they are taught the importance of asking clear, precise, and courteously phrased questions in the medical interview. Following such a practice enables them—as students and later as practicing physicians—to obtain a reliable medical history, which ultimately will be turned to the benefit of the patient by providing a basis for diagnosis and treatment. In addition, trust is fostered in and respect is shown to the patient by establishing clear and effective communication at the beginning of and throughout the patient-physician relationship.

While the transmission of moral belief is often implicit in customs and practices, the moral instruction of the physician has at times been undertaken quite explicitly as an indispensible feature of medical education. Two prominent historical examples from the eighteenth century are Dr. Benjamin Rush of Philadelphia and Dr. Samuel Bard of New York. Although Rush and Bard are not frequently mentioned today in the lecture halls and clinics of our medical schools, their writings deserve a more thorough inspection than they have recently received. Dr. Rush was one of the founders of the Philadelphia Dispensary (one of the first medical schools in the country) and wrote the first American book on psychiatry. He was active in the American Revolution and signed the Declaration of Independence for Pennsylvania. Dr. Bard, who was also active in the Revolution, helped to found what has become Columbia University's College of Physicians and Surgeons and wrote a book on diphtheria that became a classic work. These distinguished physicians and medical educators delivered formal lectures on medical ethics that were subsequently published and widely read. In his writings, Rush discusses numerous moral problems in medicine and attempts to develop elementary moral rules for medical practice—e.g., "Make it a rule never to be angry at any thing a sick man says to you. Sickness often adds to the natural impatience and irritability of the temper."[12] Bard identifies duties and virtues that serve as a strong "coun-

---

[12]Benjamin Rush, *Observations on the Duties of a Physician and the Methods of Improving Medicine, Accommodated to the Present Society and Manner in the United States.* Delivered in the University of Pennsylvania, 7 February 1789, at the conclusion of a course of lectures upon chemistry and the practice of physic. Published at the request of the class (Philadelphia: Pritchard & Hall, 1789), p. 30.

terpoise to self-interest."[13] He thus brings medical ethics close to broader conceptions of the moral person.[14]

The overall *purpose* or *object* of our institutions or morality, as transmitted by many different sources, is debatable, but a reasonable hypothesis (which we construct largely from the writings of the eighteenth-century philosopher David Hume[15] and the twentieth-century philosopher G. J. Warnock[16]) is the following: Morality ameliorates the tendency for things to go wrong or badly in interpersonal human relationships. Conditions can seriously deteriorate in human affairs as a result of limited resources, limited time, limited information, and, most important, limited sympathies. Given these pervasive features of the human condition, moral guides are needed in a culture to counter the limited human sympathies that can lead to unfortunate and even tragic situations, especially if self-interest becomes dominant in human relationships.

This analysis also suffices as an account of the purpose of the institution of medical ethics. Moral principles and action-guides counter limited sympathies, which can hamper the encounter between physician and patient. Moral principles function to keep things from going badly in the important interpersonal relationships intrinsic to medical practice by directing the physician to duties and virtues that promote the *patient's* best interests, rather than the physician's own personal interests.

Principled Philosophical Reasoning

In the midst of this cultural milieu of rules and limited sympathies, philosophers contribute as much clarity, substance, and precision of argument as can be introduced in the moral life. To this end, philosophers critically examine the corpus of writings on medical ethics and bring ethical theory to bear on moral responsibility in medicine. They seek to put medical ethics into a more unified and defensible shape than its initial cultural forms possess.

---

[13]Samuel Bard, *A Discourse upon the Duties of a Physician with Some Sentiments on the Usefulness and Necessity of a Public Hospital: Delivered before the President and Governors of King's College at the Commencement Held on the 16th of May, 1769, as Advice to Those Gentlemen Who then Received the First Medical Degrees Conferred by That University* (New York: A & J Robertson, 1969), p. 9.

[14]Similar injunctions, however, do appear in contemporary medical literature. They emphasize the importance of training medical students and physicians to examine their own attitudes and feelings and to appreciate the significance to the patient of the physician's words and behavior. See, for example, Sharon Guild and Meyer Gunther, "Patient Perspectives Program: A Humanistic Educational Experience for Medical Students," *Archives of Physical and Rehabilitation Medicine* 62 (September 1981): 461–66; and Thomas C. Fleming, "Communications," *Postgraduate Medicine* 70 (October 1981): 13–14.

[15]David Hume, *A Treatise of Human Nature*, ed. L. A. Selby-Bigge, 2d ed. rev. P. H. Nidditch (Oxford: Oxford University Press, 1978), Book III.

[16] G. J. Warnock, *The Object of Morality* (London: Methuen and Co., 1971), pp. 15–23, 71–86.

The currently favored language to express this ambition centers on "justification": Philosophers seek a reasoned defense for a system of norms of conduct from a comprehensive and coherent moral point of view. Through the medium of moral principles, philosophers try to distinguish a good moral claim—one that can be justified in terms of principles—from a bad moral claim—one that cannot be justified in terms of principles. To this end, philosophers try to exhibit how not to confuse a merely personal attitude or intuition—i.e., unreflective and nonobjective "principles"—with a reasoned and justified moral position. One must have defensible moral reasons for holding a position, and neither the position nor the reasons that underlie it can be justified if they rest solely on prejudice, emotion, false data, the authority of another individual, or claims of self-evidence. This matter is crucial because the moral principles provide reasons for action that transcend the particular beliefs of individual physicians.

In order to implement this approach, we shall focus on models of moral responsibility in medicine: frameworks that show how the physician's obligations and virtues are derived from moral principles. Philosophers appeal to a number of moral principles such as justice, liberty, respect for autonomy, equal treatment, beneficence, and utility. As we shall see in the next chapter, two moral principles are essential in medical ethics: the principle of beneficence (one should provide benefits and prevent or remove harms to others), and the principle of respect for autonomy (one should regard others as rightly self-governing). There are both philosophical and historical reasons for appealing to these principles. Because they express in distinctive ways the moral significance of promoting the best interests of the patient, we shall argue that both are required to express the physician's responsibilities to patients.

Dr. Worthington Hooker, a Connecticut physician who played a prominent role in advancing the fledgling American Medical Association, provides a classical and also controversial example of the use of the moral principle of beneficence in medicine. He argues that the physician must be truthful to patients and avoid deceiving them, even if the deception is for their benefit:

> I think it perfectly evident, that the good, which may be done by deception in a *few* cases, is almost as nothing, compared with the evil which it does in *many* cases, when the prospect of its doing good was just as promising as it was in those in which it succeeded. And when we add to this the evil which would result from a *general* adoption of a system of deception, the importance of a strict adherence to truth in our intercourse with the sick, even on the ground of expedience, becomes incalculably great.[17]

---

[17]Worthington Hooker, *Physician and Patient* (New York: Baker and Scribner, 1849), in *Ethics in Medicine,* ed. Stanley Reiser et al., p. 211.

Most writers who defend nondeception in medical disclosures appeal to the principle of respect for the autonomy of patients, but Hooker appeals to an analysis of the harm to patients that deception engenders, based on his prediction of the consequences of a practice of deception in patient care.

Criteria of Philosophical Reasoning

Moral principles are best defended in philosophy in the context of a full ethical theory. While we cannot here outline in detail the nature of philosophical theories, there are widely agreed upon criteria of philosophical reasoning about morality that govern moral justification. These criteria explicate what is meant by such expressions as "reasoned discourse about morals."

The first criterion is *clarity*. When physicians like Dr. Hildreth must make decisions about whether it is consistent with their moral responsibilities to patients to allow a newborn infant to die, they must deal with vagueness and possible confusion.[18] For example, distinctions such as that between killing and allowing to die[19] can determine the outcome of their deliberations. Yet these distinctions are often vague and deserve careful analysis and clarification of their roles in moral thinking. We demand clarity so that basic concepts will be as free from equivocation and ambiguity as possible. Only then can "clear-headed" moral thinking occur. In Dr. Hildreth's case study, for example, some concepts are reasonably clear, but the central concept of "mental life" goes unexamined. Such an important concept requires further explication if we are to be free of crippling confusions in such contexts. A major task for us in this book is to express clearly the meaning of "the patient's best interests," which in turn establishes the meaning of the injunction to promote the patient's best interests.

The second criterion of philosophical reasoning is *consistency*. A specific belief that a physician might have—e.g., a belief about allowing infants with serious birth defects to die—could be inconsistent with other beliefs he or she intuitively holds, such as that patients in respiratory distress should always be resuscitated. Consistency requires that contradiction be avoided in our reasoning. For example, the widely quoted, allegedly traditional principle of medical ethics, "Do no harm," can easily lead to contradictory imperatives about the disclosure of information to seriously or terminally ill patients. It can demand that the truth be told in order to avoid harm (as Hooker argues) and that the truth be withheld in order to avoid harm (as we shall witness several physicians arguing in chapter three). This possibil-

---

[18]Anthony Shaw, Judson G. Randolph, and Barbara Manard, "Ethical Issues in Pediatric Surgery: A National Survey of Pediatricians and Pediatric Surgeons," *Pediatrics* 60 (Pt. 2: October, 1977): 588–99.

[19]James Rachels, "Active and Passive Euthanasia," *The New England Journal of Medicine* 292 (9 January 1975): 78–80.

ity suggests the need for a more elaborate formulation of the conditions under which disclosures do and do not cause harm, a formulation that renders the principle and its application consistent.[20]

Clarity and consistency will aid us throughout this volume in the attempt to improve upon and critically analyze law and morality. However, use of these criteria will not resolve all our problems. Moral principles may still pull us in different directions in specific cases. Ethical theory introduces clarity and consistency, but not perfect outcomes. Philosophical ethics can no more be expected to lead in straight and uncomplicated lines to the resolution of moral problems than can traditional writings in medical ethics. Two clear and consistent lines of philosophical reasoning, based in different principles, can fall into conflict, and seemingly irresolvable moral controversies may result. This difficulty leads us to the subject of conflicting moral principles, a central problem for philosophical ethics and medical ethics alike.

PRINCIPLES, DUTIES, AND VIRTUES

The theme of many a successful novel and film centers on how obligations based in different principles of duty come into conflict in the moral life. For example, an impoverished person may steal in order to preserve a life, a soldier may lie in order to protect a sworn secret, or a physician may break confidentiality in order to protect a person endangered by its maintenance. In each case, it must be decided which (if either) moral obligation has priority over the moral obligation with which it conflicts—e.g., whether the obligation that physicians not violate patient confidences is to be given priority, in certain circumstances, over the obligation that physicians should protect the lives of innocent persons endangered by patients. How to weigh and balance one moral obligation against another is a major task of moral reasoning.

Prima Facie Duties

In a classic analysis of this task, the Oxford philosopher W. D. Ross has developed a theory of "*prima facie* duties."[21] Ross argues that there are several different sources and types of moral duties. For example, our prom-

---

[20]Consistency also requires that whenever we judge an act under a certain description to be right (or wrong), we are logically committed to judging all relevantly similar acts under the same description right (or wrong) for any person in similar circumstances. The rules apply to everyone *relevantly situated,* although the rules might not apply to someone in quite different circumstances. This is one component in Dr. Hooker's argument.

[21]W. D. Ross, *The Right and the Good* (Oxford: Oxford University Press, 1930), p. 19ff. Some valuable warnings about the interpretation of Ross's notion of a prima facie duty are found in John Searle, "Prima Facie Obligations," in Joseph Raz, ed., *Practical Reasoning* (Oxford: Oxford University Press, 1978), pp. 81–90; and John Atwell, "Ross and Prima Facie Duties," *Ethics* 88 (1978): 240–49.

ises create duties of fidelity, wrongful actions create duties of reparation, and the generous gifts of our friends create duties of gratitude. Ross lists other principles of duty as well, such as those of self-improvement, nonmaleficence, beneficence, and justice. According to Ross, we must find "the greatest duty" in any given circumstance by finding "the greatest balance" of right over wrong in the particular context. Ross then introduces his central distinction between *prima facie* duties and *actual* duties: "Prima facie duty" refers to a duty always to be acted upon unless it conflicts on a particular occasion with an equal or stronger duty. A prima facie duty, we might say, is always right and binding, all other things being equal. While it is a firm duty, it is nonetheless conditional on not being overridden or outweighed by competing moral demands. One's actual duty is determined by an examination of the respective weights of the competing prima facie duties.

Consider, as an example, a case we shall discuss in chapter four: A seventy-three-year-old man was mortally ill in a hospital and required a mechanical respirator. He had been judged competent, but his request to have the respirator disconnected was refused. He then attempted to disconnect it himself. The matter wound up in court. The patient contended that, in the face of his misery, the hospital and his physicians had an obligation to allow him to make his own choices, even though his choice entailed his death. His physicians and legal representatives of the state of Florida argued that they had a duty to preserve life and to prevent suicide. Here the duty to preserve life is in direct conflict with the duty to respect the autonomy of another person. Both are prima facie duties. A Florida court then had to fix the actual duty of the hospital and physicians. In a complicated balancing of the conflicting obligations, the court argued that the patient's choice should be overriding because considerations of autonomy were *here* (though not *everywhere*) weightier. The court reasoned that in this case "the cost to the individual" of refusing to recognize his choice in a circumstance of terminal illness could not be overridden by the duty to preserve life.[22]

Beneficence and Respect for Autonomy

Ross may be correct in holding that there are *many* distinct prima facie moral duties, each expressible in terms of a moral principle that grounds or generates the duty. However, as already noted, in this book we shall emphasize *two* principles as having paramount importance for medical ethics: *respect for autonomy* and *beneficence*. Respect for autonomy is a principle requiring that we regard others as rightfully self-governing (autonomous) in matters of their choice and action, whereas beneficence requires us to

[22]*Satz v. Perlmutter*, 362 So.2d 160 (Florida District Court of Appeals, 1978), 379 So.2d (Florida, 1980).

provide positive benefits as well as to prevent and remove harmful conditions.

In contrast to certain writers in medical ethics who hold that the physician's responsibility for the autonomous patient can be explained by reference to the principle of autonomy alone, we shall argue that respect for autonomy is a prima facie principle; therefore, it has no more than a prima facie claim to override the principle of beneficence when the two conflict. With Ross, we defend the view that neither respect for autonomy nor any one moral principle has sufficient weight to trump all conflicting moral claims. The metaphor of weights moving up and down on a balance scale has often been criticized as out of place and as potentially misleading in its apparent simplicity, and this is a caution we all should heed. However, philosophers have yet to provide a more adequate way of formulating the problem of conflicting principles, and our analysis in subsequent chapters presupposes that *a pluralism of (a priori) equally weighted moral principles* is a fundamental feature of the moral life generally and of the moral life in medicine in particular.

We can again turn to truth-telling as an excellent example of a problem that often involves reference to both beneficence and respect for autonomy as grounds of the physician's actual duty. On the one hand, the physician must give weight to the patient's right to know (because the principle of autonomy demands it) and must also give weight to the possible harmful effects of keeping a patient ignorant (because, as Hooker argues, the principle of beneficence demands it). On the other hand, weight must be given to the obligation not to alarm the fragile or seriously ill patient (because, again, the principle of beneficence demands it). To argue, as many have, that not telling patients the truth is "prima facie wrong" means simply that an act that involves withholding information is wrong if there is no moral justification for the withholding. But if there *is* a sufficient justification, based on a principle having greater weight *in the circumstances*, then one can validly withhold the information.

Consider the position taken by Dr. Bard. Anticipating Dr. Hooker's later views, Bard held, in 1769, that there is a strong obligation to be truthful to the dying patient. Deception, he argues, "is really cruel, as the stroke of death is always most severely felt, when unexpected; and the grim tyrant may in general be disarmed of his terrors, and rendered familiar to the most timid, and apprehensive." Moreover, Bard contends, "those to whom the thoughts of death are painful, are too apt when flattered with the prospect of recovery, to neglect the necessary provision against a disappointment, and by that means involve their families in confusion and distress."[23] For Bard, the physician's actual duty is almost always to disclose the prediction of impending death, because the harms to be avoided for

---

[23]Bard, *A Discourse Upon the Duties of a Physician*, p. 11.

the patient and his family almost always outweigh those of fright and anxiety that might be caused by such a disclosure.

Nevertheless, if some more weighty moral consideration, such as protecting the fragile patient from harm, happens to prevail in particular circumstances, the physician may be obligated to withhold information temporarily. This is the approach taken to the moral problem of truth-telling by Richard Clarke Cabot, a Boston physician and Harvard professor at the beginning of our century. Taking much the same view as Dr. Hooker, Cabot argues that "A straight answer to a straight question is what I am recommending, not an unasked presentation of any of the facts of the patient's case. . . . But a straight answer does not mean what is often called the 'blunt truth,' the 'naked truth,' the dry cold facts. Veracity means . . . the attempt to convey a true impression, a fully drawn and properly shaded account such as is, as I well know, very difficult to give."[24] Cabot proposes that we ought (prima facie) to tell the truth, but that we ought (prima facie) to protect other interests of the patient as well. The physician is constantly confronted by such conflicting demands. Cabot resolves the conflict in favor of the actual duty to be honest in all disclosures to patients, but to time the sequence of disclosure so that the patient is not unnecessarily harmed.

This brief review of historical arguments about truth-telling leads to a central thesis that Ross also advances: No moral philosopher has ever been able to present a system of moral rules free of these kinds of conflicts between principles and exceptions to principles. Ross argues that the nature of the moral life itself makes an exception-free hierarchy of rules and principles impossible. This thesis has strong appeal, even though the metaphor of the "weight" of a principle of duty has not proven amenable to precise analysis. Ross's thesis covers circumstances where a *single* principle directs us to two equally attractive alternatives, only one of which can be pursued, as in applications of the principle of beneficence to problems of truth-telling to patients. Whether the conflict is of this sort or between two different principles, there may not be a *single* right action in some circumstances, because there may be *two* or *more* morally acceptable actions unavoidably in conflict.

Moral Virtues and Moral Character

Moral obligations, expressed through principles of duty, are not the whole of morality, and we make as many assessments of the moral *character* of persons as we do of their *obligations*. We speak of physicians, and indeed all persons, as having good or bad characters and as exhibiting certain virtues and certain vices. For this reason, philosophical ethics examines both obli-

---

[24]Richard C. Cabot, "The Use of Truth and Falsehood in Medicine," *American Medicine* 5 (1903): 344–49, in *Ethics in Medicine*, ed. Stanley Reiser et al., pp. 217–18.

gations and virtues. Virtues are well-established dispositions or habits to do what is morally commendable. Such habits or traits of character are of major importance in the hurried context of medical practice. The goal of cultivating virtues is to make the fulfillment of duties to patients a matter of established behavior, rather than a constant struggle to enforce the demands of moral principles.

An ethics of virtue involves an assessment of selected traits of character such as honesty, tactfulness, and trustworthiness. Such traits establish a person's moral character. Most people have a moral character that varies over time in its strength and predictability, but even when variation results (e.g., from occasional moral weakness or ill health), we tend to retain our view of a person's typical moral behavior. We say, for example, that some choices arising from momentary desires do not represent the person faithfully because they do not express well-established preferences and beliefs. A person may, of course, be of virtuous character in some respects (e.g., possessing conscientiousness and trustworthiness), while suffering from deficiencies in other respects (e.g., lacking in patience and tolerance).

In ethical theory, moral virtues are generally, and perhaps always, *correlated* with moral principles of duty.[25] That is, for every moral principle, such as beneficence and respect for autonomy, there corresponds one or more moral virtues or dispositions to act in accordance with the duties derived from the principle—e.g., virtues of benevolence and respectfulness. In order to know which virtues are appropriate in medicine, we need first to know what *ought* to be done, and a theory of moral principles of duty presumably provides such an account of what ought to be done. Thus, in moral theory, a study of the virtues is integrally tied to an examination of proper moral principles and the duties they generate. The language of virtues buttresses, rather than *supplants,* the language of principles of duty[26] because both duties and virtues are required to make moral responsibility a "counterpoise to self-interest" and thus to direct the physician to the best interests of the patient.

A number of major figures in the history of medical ethics emphasize the virtues of the physician. One of the most important of these was Thomas Percival, a physician living in Manchester, England, at the end of the eighteenth century. His book, *Medical Ethics* (1803), opens with the following

[25]Many virtues such as kindness, generosity, and affection may express ideals rather than duties, and so may not correspond to duties.

[26]This account of moral virtue is similar to that of Gregory Pence, who holds that virtue involves "having such a character that one *wants* to do the morally right act" and not simply because duty *forces* one to do so. See his *Ethical Options in Medicine* (Oradell, N.J.: Medical Economics Company, Book Division, 1980), p. 25. See also Alasdair MacIntyre's depiction: "A virtue is an acquired human quality the possession and exercise of which tends to enable us to achieve those goals which are internal to practices and the lack of which effectively prevents us from achieving any such goods." *After Virtue* (Notre Dame, Ind.: University of Notre Dame Press, 1981), p. 178.

admonition: "Hospital physicians and surgeons should minister to the sick, with due impressions of the importance of their office. . . . They should study, also, in their deportment, so to unite *tenderness* with *steadiness,* and *condescension* with *authority,* as to inspire the minds of their patients with gratitude, respect and confidence."[27]

Because they are jarring to the contemporary reader, words like "condescension" and "authority" tend to distort the logic of Percival's views. Yet they are extraordinarily compelling virtues of the physician in his conception. Percival moves from elementary premises about the patient's best interests being the proper object of the physician's skills to characterizations of the physician's proper deportment, including traits of character requisite to promote the patient's best interests. Condescension means, in this context, a courteous disregard or indifference on the physician's part to his own rank or standing, in deference to serving the patient. That is, recognizing the dependence of patients, physicians should put aside lofty pride and dignity. Failure to do so may distract the physician from the patient's best interests. Authority directs the physician to the fulfillment of obligations to patients, as a seasoned professional understands those obligations. Authority balances condescension by forestalling undue identification with the patient.

Percival's views had considerable influence on subsequent medical ethics. The passage above appears nearly *verbatim* in the opening lines of the first *Code of Ethics* of the American Medical Association.[28] In a book published in 1883, the American physician Austin Flint interpreted the intentions of the authors of the AMA *Code* in much the same way as we have intepreted Percival. "The sentiments so admirably expressed in the foregoing first paragraph of the code need no arguments for their support, nor any comments to increase their force. They antagonize undue influences arising from self-conceit, an irritable temper, indolence, devotion to pleasure or to occupations *which divert us from professional duties,* and all mercenary considerations."[29]

Accounts of the virtues of physicians traditionally include reference to traits of character or habits that direct the physician away from self-interest to the fulfillment of "professional duties," including moral obligations in patient care. For example, Sir William Osler, one of the great figures of modern medicine, writes of *aequanimitas,* the "bodily" and "mental" virtue

----

[27]Percival, *Percival's Medical Ethics,* p. 71.

[28]The language in the first AMA *Code of Ethics* is the following: "They should study, also, in their deportment, so to unite *tenderness* with *firmness,* and *condescension* with *authority,* as to inspire the minds of their patients with gratitude, respect, and confidence." American Medical Association, *Proceedings of the National Medical Convention 1846–1847,* in *Ethics in Medicine,* ed. Stanley Reiser et al., p. 29.

[29]Austin Flint, Sr., *Medical Ethics and Etiquette: The Code of Ethics Adopted by the American Medical Association, with Commentaries* (New York: D. Appleton and Company, 1883), p. 8 (emphasis added).

of "imperturbability."[30] Exploring the ramifications of this trait of character for professional life and practice, Osler urges physicians to be steady in the face of medical uncertainty and to have courage in the face of failure. Acquiring such traits or habits will assist the physician to maintain "mental equilibrium" without at the same time "hardening 'the human heart by which we all live'."[31] Through acquiring and practicing the virtue of *aequanimitas,* the physician becomes a professional in a basic sense: one who is devoted in a disciplined, reliable, and humane manner to those under one's care.

Attention to such virtues as *aequanimitas* is no mere historical curiosity or relic. There is a persistent emphasis on the virtues of the physician in contemporary medical literature. In the specific area of the care of cancer patients, for instance, some writers have identified a composite picture of the physician "who possesses desirable, affective characteristics relative to cancer management," with a special emphasis on "compassion with cancer patients."[32] The importance of the virtue of empathy has also found frequent defense.[33]

Finally, a study of the virtues can be important because of their expression of a character that *exceeds* moral obligations. Sympathy, generosity, tact, and the like are extremely important in the life of the physician, even under conditions not in any strict sense required by duty. It has often been asserted in the history of medical ethics that the best physician, and the one to be cultivated and sought out, is the kind, discerning, sympathetic, determined, and patient person. We shall find numerous occasions on which to test this hypothesis.

Challenging Traditional Presuppositions

Despite our emphasis on history, traditional moral beliefs, established duties, and cultural contexts, it should not be overlooked that philosophy at its best involves careful and critical reflection on what people often take for granted. One of the major functions of philosophy in every period has been to challenge fundamental cultural presuppositions. For example, a deep assumption of our age—reflected unflinchingly in recent pronouncements of the American Medical Association—is that active killing of patients cannot be condoned in medicine under any circumstances.[34] Similarly we tend to believe that to treat someone who is not a child

[30]William Osler, "Aequanimitas," in *Aequanimitas: With Other Addresses to Medical Students, Nurses, and Practitioners of Medicine* (Philadelphia: P. Blakiston's Son and Co., 1904).

[31]Ibid., 5.

[32]Edwin Barnes et al., "Faculty and House Staff Attitudes Toward Cancer: Status and Comparison," *Journal of Medical Education* 57 (January 1982): 48–53.

[33]See, for example, Ursula Streit-Forest, "Differences in Empathy: A Preliminary Analysis," *Journal of Medical Education* 57 (January 1982): 65–67.

[34]See Rachels, "Active and Passive Euthanasia," 78–80.

paternalistically is to treat the person wrongly. While these and many other traditonal assumptions *may* turn out to be well founded, it is part of the role of philosophy to challenge such assumptions and not to be satisfied until they have been thoroughly defended by good reasons. Regrettably, philosophers themselves often forget this role, for they are as much a part of their cultures as anyone else. This is important in the present context because many moral problems in medicine require us to revise traditional ways of handling them. Sometimes we are challenged to cast aside assumptions that deeply predispose us to one alternative rather than another, and we come out better for having accepted the challenge.

THE REMAINDER OF THIS VOLUME

"To the trained eye," writes Dr. Norman Fost, "*every* patient presents an ethical problem."[35] From decisions about whether to discuss the risks of aspirin to whether a parent should be told that a medical student or intern is performing his or her first procedure on a child, the discerning physician will know that even the most routine dimensions of medicine permit no escape from moral problems. In subsequent chapters we shall dwell no less on these dimensions of medicine than on dramatic encounters with patients such as Dr. Hildreth's. The arguments in these subsequent chapters are erected on the historical and philosophical foundations established in this chapter. A major theme of this first chapter has been that there are problems about how to apply and "weight" moral principles. This view of prima facie principles is used in chapter two to build two basic models of moral responsibility that are essential for medical ethics. These models provide philosophical frameworks that translate "promoting the patient's best interests" into concrete moral responsibilities of physicians.

The two moral principles that underlie these models are beneficence and respect for autonomy. The first model we therefore call the "beneficence model." It has its principal roots in the history of medical ethics. The second model, the "autonomy model," has its principal roots in the histories of philosophy and Anglo-American law. Because the models embrace distinctive perspectives on the best interests of patients, and thus distinctive principles of duty, they sometimes come into conflict, making a central task of medical ethics that of negotiating between competing prima facie obligations.

Chapters three through five examine how entrenched and difficult these conflicts can be in the patient-physician relationship, and how at the same time the physician's responsibilities to patients can be discharged only by discretion in balancing the moral demands of these principles. In chapter

---

[35]Norman Fost, "Ethical Problems in Pediatrics," *Current Problems in Pediatrics* 6 (October 1976): 3 (emphasis added).

six we complete our inquiry by examining the extent to which the physician should take account of obligations to third parties, obligations that may be in conflict with the physician's obligations to patients. Chapters one through six are thus connected by the theme of prima facie principles and obligations that come into conflict. The six chapters may be outlined as follows:

Chapter	Title	Purpose
1	Moral Reasoning in Medicine	To examine moral reasoning in medicine, with an emphasis on the theme of moral conflict in discharging responsibilities.
2	Two Models of Moral Responsibility in Medicine	To introduce two models of moral responsibility in medicine: the beneficence model and the autonomy model.
3	The Management of Medical Information	To explore conflicts between the two models that are created by the demand to respect autonomy in disclosures of information to patients.
4	Medical Paternalism	To explore conflicts between the two models that are created by the demand to act beneficently in protecting patients from harm.
5	Reduced Autonomy and Diminished Competence	To explore, through applications of both models, obligations to patients who are compromised by illness or medical intervention.
6	Third-Party Interests	To explore conflicts between obligations to patients and obligations to third parties.

As this outline and our earlier discussion about conflict in the moral life suggest, we do not view medical ethics as dictating decisions to doctors. Instead, it provides reasoned and systematic approaches to moral problems. The resultant lack of certainty is not a matter for despair, although it certainly complicates the resolution of moral problems. Well-motivated people can disagree for rationally compelling reasons, and tolerance of views of those who disagree for principled reasons is the most compelling form of tolerance. Even if one believes another to be morally misguided, tolerance and respect are preferable to dismissal. Disagreements are sure to emerge over difficult moral problems, and their genuine resolution will usually occur only if attitudes prevail that allow for criticism and revision. Such attitudes are essential because human conduct in general, and professional conduct in particular, will never be governed with the certainties present in a system of geometry. Nonetheless, medical ethics can be written to yield clear, consistent, and reliable accounts of the moral responsibilities of physicians.

Chapter 2

Two Models
of Moral Responsibility
in Medicine

We saw in the first chapter that moral responsibility in medicine is to be understood in terms of prima facie moral principles and the duties and virtues that these principles generate. In this chapter we examine two broad models of moral responsibility that rest on these foundations. These models share a common origin in the moral purpose of promoting the best interests of the patient. Each model is developed in terms of two fundamental perspectives from which those interests can be interpreted.

The first model understands the patient's best interests exclusively from the perspective of medicine. By medicine we mean the repository of tested knowledge, skills, and experience constituting the science and art of the cure, alleviation, and prevention of disease and injury. Medicine in this sense establishes the main sources for discovering and corroborating hypotheses about health and disease, which, in turn, form the basis for diagnosis, treatment, and prognosis. So understood, medicine provides what we designate an *objective* perspective on the patient's best interests. "Objective" means simply that the perspective transcends the particular and sometimes idiosyncratic beliefs or approach of the individual physician. The goals of the medical enterprise, as well as the duties and virtues of the physician, are expressed in terms of both goods that should be sought on behalf of patients and harms to be avoided. Because the principle of beneficence expresses the moral significance of seeking the greater balance of good over harm for another, we call this the *beneficence model* of moral responsibility in medicine.

The second model interprets the best interests of the patient exclusively from the perspective of the patient, as he or she understands them. This perspective may sometimes be starkly different from that of medicine. The physician's respect for the patient's values and beliefs is the source of the duties and virtues appropriate to the second model. Because the principle of respect for autonomy expresses the moral significance of respecting another's values and beliefs, we call this the *autonomy model* of moral responsibility in medicine.

22

Models based in the utterly different commitments of the principles of beneficence and autonomy might at first glance seem to be in hopeless opposition, forcing the physician to choose one to the exclusion of the other. On closer examination this conclusion proves to be unwarranted. Each model is best viewed as capturing a valid but *partial* perspective on the responsibilities of physicians. Just as a theory of the moral life would be impoverished if it contained but a single principle, such as beneficence or respect for autonomy, so would a theory of the moral responsibilities of physicians be impoverished if but one model were accepted as the exclusive authority.[1] Medicine is enhanced and dignified by both, although, like moral principles, the two models can come into frustrating conflict. We argued in chapter one that such moral conflict is inescapable, and the two models developed in this chapter should be viewed as frameworks for clearly identifying and negotiating such moral conflict in medicine. The following case study introduces these themes.

A CASE STUDY: ELECTIVE STERILIZATION

Elizabeth Monroe is a twenty-six-year-old woman, a nonsmoker in excellent health. She has just completed her doctoral degree in physics and will soon start a two-year postdoctoral fellowship to do further work in her special area of interest, high-energy physics, after which she intends to seek an academic position. She was divorced one year ago, ending a very trying marriage that lasted only two years. There were no children from the marriage and Ms. Monroe has never been pregnant. She has been taking birth control pills for the past six years without any complications.

Dr. Regina Cox has been Ms. Monroe's gynecologist for the past five years. At her regular visit, after Dr. Cox has completed the physical examination, she asks Ms. Monroe if she has any questions or other matters about her health that she would like to discuss. Ms. Monroe is forthright: She asks Dr. Cox to perform a tubal ligation, a procedure that severs the oviducts and leaves a woman unable to conceive.

Dr. Cox responds that sterilization is a serious matter and that she would like to discuss with Ms. Monroe both the procedure and her reasons for

---

[1]Allan Crimm and Raymond Greenberg, both physicians, criticize the single model approach in their "Reflections on the Doctor-Patient Relationship," in *Ethical Dimensions of Clinical Medicine*, ed. Dennis A. Robbins and Allen R. Dyer (Springfield, Ill.: Charles C Thomas, Publisher, 1981), pp. 104–10. See also David C. Thomasma, "Limitations of the Autonomy Model for the Doctor-Patient Relationship," *The Pharos* (Spring 1983): 2–5.

wanting it performed. A tubal ligation is performed via laparoscopy[2] to cauterize[3] the oviducts. This procedure can be performed under a local anesthetic, which involves fewer risks than general anesthesia. The long-run risks of tubal ligation itself are not known, but there is some evidence that there may be changes in prostaglandin levels.[4] These consequences, however, are not regarded as significant health risks.

For someone of Ms. Monroe's age and health status, then, laparoscopy poses minimal risk, as do the consequences of sterilization. In addition, a woman of her age with a history free of complications in the use of the pill, and who is not a smoker, does not face significant risks in continuing on birth control pills (even for another eight or nine years). Indeed, recent studies indicate that women like Ms. Monroe may actually experience benefits from the pill, including possible prevention of various forms of cancer.[5]

Dr. Cox explains these facts in some detail and then asks Ms. Monroe if she has considered alternative methods of birth control, e.g., the implantation of an intrauterine device (IUD). Ms. Monroe says that the IUD was the first form of birth control she tried, during her college years. She experienced problems with bleeding and gave up the IUD. Because other forms of birth control were not as effective as the pill, she switched to it when she was twenty.

Dr. Cox then asks whether Ms. Monroe has thought about the possibility of marriage to a man who may want to have children. Ms. Monroe replies that she would like to marry again, but that she definitely does not want to have children. Her ex-husband, she says, wanted to have children, and her decision not to be a parent was a source of stress in their marriage and was a major reason for their divorce. She says that she will surely be more careful in any possible future marriage to discuss thoroughly a prospective husband's attitudes about having children. If he should want children, then she would definitely not marry him, as painful as that decision might turn out to be.

Ms. Monroe replies that she has thought about this matter at length, especially in light of her experience with marriage. She says that she is deeply

---

[2]Laparoscopy is a procedure involving the insertion through a surgical incision of a laparoscope, a flexible tube, to view the abdominal contents and to perform limited surgical procedures.

[3]Cauterization is a procedure involving the severing of vessels, in this case the fallopian tubes, by burning, as a means to seal the wound and speed healing.

[4]Prostaglandins are chemicals released in various parts of the body, changes in which are associated with such health problems as heart disease.

[5]B. S. Hulka et al., "Protection Against Endometrial Carcinoma by Combination-Product Oral Contraceptives," *Journal of the American Medical Association* 247 (22–29 January 1982): 475–77; and "Oral Contraceptives and Cancer Risk," *Morbidity and Mortality Weekly Report* 31 (30 July 1982): 393–94.

dedicated to her scientific work, which is the most important thing in her life and which therefore absorbs most of her energy and interest. She is excited about her future study and research in high-energy physics. She enthusiastically recounts that it is a demanding field and that, if she is to make a significant contribution in research and teaching, she will have to work even harder than she did in graduate school. Because of these career demands, she says, she would not have the time required for children. She would not welcome the interruptions child-bearing and child-rearing would bring to her career, and she believes little time could be devoted to caring for children. For these reasons she does not want to have children.

Dr. Cox then suggests to Ms. Monroe that she may change her mind about children after a few years. Dr. Cox recounts a piece of her personal history: When she was in her late twenties she felt almost exactly like Ms. Monroe about her career and lifestyle. However, over the years she met the "right man" and had two children. Now she is forty-eight and her two children are at the center of her life. Ms. Monroe replies that she thinks that such a change in her plans is unlikely. She has spent the last several months, she says, thinking through these issues. She has made up her mind only after carefully weighing the pros and cons of sterilization and testing her ideas in extensive conversations with other women scientists. She reiterates that she wants a *permanent* means of birth control.

She tells Dr. Cox that in a month she is due for a two-week vacation before she commences her postdoctoral studies. She wants to be worked-up in the intervening time and requests that Dr. Cox schedule her for the procedure at the beginning of her vacation.

Ms. Monroe is an unusually well informed and thoughtful patient. She has taken the time to explore the benefits and health risks of various contraceptive techniques. As a scientist, she is presumably capable of understanding the complex nature of those benefits and risks. Moreover, she has arrived at her decision for sterilization after lengthy and thoughtful deliberation. Hers is not a rash or impulsive request. Indeed, it is autonomous and well informed.

How should Dr. Cox respond to Ms. Monroe's request for sterilization? Here, Dr. Cox's realistic alternatives seem to be the following: (1) She can refuse to perform the sterilization on grounds that it is not in Ms. Monroe's best interests, as medicine understands those interests. (2) She can refuse to perform the sterilization on grounds that Ms. Monroe's decision is not acceptable to her as an individual. (3) Dr. Cox can perform the sterilization as requested, because it is in Ms. Monroe's best interests, as her patient understands those interests. The arguments supporting each response draw in distinctive ways on the beneficence and autonomy models.

MODELS OF MORAL RESPONSIBILITY

Before considering each model in detail, the meaning of a "model" must be clarified. We use this term in ways analogous to the literature on models of the patient-physician relationship in general, but ours is confined to moral responsibilities in that relationship. Consider for example, the models proposed by Drs. Thomas Szasz and Marc Hollender in their classic article,[6] as well as the "biopsychosocial model" proposed by Dr. George Engel.[7] These models are designed to permit the physician both to analyze and to direct his or her behavior in patient care. Szasz's and Hollender's model of guidance-cooperation, for example, helps the physician deal with the patient who is temporarily distracted by anxiety or fear and who may therefore need to be "guided" for a time until his or her decisions can be free of such distractions. At that point another model comes into play, that of mutual participation, which directs the physician to treat the patient as an equal. Engel's model helps the physician to appreciate nonbiological factors that influence illness, such as the patient's family, occupation, and ethnic or cultural traditions. In addition, the biopsychosocial model directs the physician to identify how psychosocial factors affect the patient's recovery so that their impact on the patient's health can be controlled, or at least ameliorated.

The two models that we develop aid the physician in analyzing and justifying morally appropriate physician attitudes and behavior in patient care. In the case of Ms. Monroe's request for a sterilization procedure, as we shall see, each model helps the physician to interpret the moral significance of Ms. Monroe's request. Each also directs the physician to particular obligations and virtues. The perspective each model takes is expressed in terms of a moral principle that generates those obligations and virtues.

We use the language of *models* (rather than *principles*) to convey the idea of a complex pattern that shows the arrangement of its parts—like, for example, an architect's model. The verb "to model" can also mean "to give shape to" and "to make a tool of." In developing these models we are giving shape to what is only inchoate and unsystematically formed in medical practice, as well as in the history of medical ethics. We are simultaneously

---

[6]Thomas S. Szasz and Marc H. Hollender, "A Contribution to the Philosophy of Medicine: The Basic Models of the Doctor-Patient Relationship," *Archives of Internal Medicine* 97 (1956): 585–92.

[7]George L. Engel, "The Need for a New Medical Model: A Challenge for Biomedicine," *Science* 196 (1977): 129–36; "The Biopsychosocial Model and the Education of Health Professionals," *Annals of the New York Academy of Science* 310 (1978): 169–81; and "The Clinical Application of the Biopsychosocial Model," *American Journal of Psychiatry* 137 (1980): 535–44.

forming a tool useful in clinical practice. A mere abstract theoretical model would scarcely serve our practical objectives.[8]

Each model embraces four interconnected elements:

1. The general *moral end* of medicine: to promote the patient's best interests;
2. A *principle* that provides the moral significance of distinct perspectives on the patient's best interests;
3. *Obligations* (or duties) that derive from this principle; and
4. *Virtues* that derive from this principle.

Because they are the heart of each model, the principles of beneficence and respect for autonomy receive most of our attention in this and in subsequent chapters. Through applications of the two models, we give these abstract philosophical principles a content adapted to the clinical setting.

THE BENEFICENCE MODEL

The word "beneficence" is broadly used in English. Its meanings include the doing of good, the active promotion of good, kindness, and charity. However, any principle specifying the duty of beneficence will have a narrower meaning. In its most general form, a broadly formulated principle of beneficence requires that one help others further important and legitimate interests and abstain from injuring them.[9] But whose interests count? The principle of beneficence is clearly not restricted in its application in medical ethics to the patient-physician relationship. Because third parties to that relationship can be harmed if the physician always acts excusively to benefit his or her patient, there may be obligations of beneficence to third parties. We discuss such obligations in chapter six.[10]

---

[8]For accounts of other pertinent models in the medical ethics literature, see John Arras and Robert Hunt, eds., *Ethical Issues in Modern Medicine*, 2d ed. (Palo Alto, Calif.: Mayfield Publishing Co., 1983), Part One, Section I, which includes Robert M. Veatch's influential essay, "Models for Ethical Medicine in a Revolutionary Age," *Hastings Center Report* 2 (1972): 5–7; President's Commission for the Study of Ethical Problems in Medicine and Biomedical and Behavioral Research, *Making Health Care Decisions* (Washington, D.C.: U.S. Government Printing Office, 1982), pp. 36–39; Gregory Pence, *Ethical Options in Medicine* (Oradell, N.J.: Medical Economics Company, Book Division, 1980), pp. 185–221; and Albert R. Jonsen, Mark Siegler, and William Winslade, *Clinical Ethics* (New York: Macmillan Publishing Company, 1982), pp. 11–50.

[9]See Earl Shelp, "To Benefit and Respect Persons: A Challenge for Beneficence in Health Care," in *Beneficence and Health Care*, ed. Earl Shelp (Dordrecht, Holland: D. Reidel Publishing Co., 1982), pp. 200–204; and Tom L. Beauchamp and James Childress, *Principles of Biomedical Ethics*, 2d ed. (New York: Oxford University Press, 1983), Chapters 4–5.

[10]See also Natalie Abrams, "Scope of Beneficence in Health Care," in *Beneficence and Health Care*, ed. Earl Shelp, pp. 183–98, esp. pp. 193–97.

Many similar disputes in ethical theory concern the exact content and justification of "the principle of beneficence."[11] However, these problems need not delay us, because our overriding interest is in providing an account of the principle of beneficence that establishes its relevance for clinical practice. The central question for beneficence within the patient-physician relationship is "What does it mean for the physician to seek the greater balance of good over harm in the care of patients?" The beneficence model answers this question in terms of the perspective that medicine takes on the patient's best interests. That perspective gives the principle of beneficence specific clinically oriented meanings that define the goods and harms to be balanced. Because this perspective cannot be adequately understood if torn from its historical roots, we rely on historical writings and practices as a major source for the elements of the beneficence model.

The primary historical sources of the beneficence model of moral responsibility are found in Western medical ethics developed over the past 2,500 years. We feature but two historical periods in our analysis. The first is ancient Greece and the Hippocratic physicians who represent the tradition of oaths and codes. The undeniable importance of the Hippocratic Oath and related writings dictate this starting point. The second historical period is eighteenth-century Great Britain, in particular the medical ethics of the distinguished Scottish physician, John Gregory. Gregory's considerable influence on major events in the history of medical ethics in the nineteenth century, as well as philosophy's influence on Gregory, make him an ideal choice.

Ancient Sources of the Model

The earliest expression of the beneficence model of moral responsibility in medicine is found in the influential Hippocratic writings,[12] whose distinctive features are influential to the present day.[13] The Hippocratic

---

[11]For many important issues, see Allen Buchanan, "Philosophical Foundations of Beneficence," in *Beneficence and Health Care*, ed. Earl Shelp, pp. 33–62. Because beneficence potentially demands excessive generosity in the moral life, some philosophers have argued that it is *ideal*, but not a *duty*, to act beneficently. They view beneficent actions as approximating acts of charity, acts of conscience, or acts done from personal ideals of conduct beyond the call of duty. We shall hold, however, that beneficence is, within certain limits, a duty. Role responsibilities in medicine clearly indicate that the physician is morally obligated on at least some occasions to assist patients and to abstain from harming them. We shall give specific content to this abstract principle as we proceed—starting with the content it has traditionally been given in the history of medicine.

[12]W. H. S. Jones, trans. *Hippocrates* (Cambridge: Harvard University Press, the Loeb Classical Library, 1923).

[13]For an analysis of these features, see Ludwig Edelstein, *Ancient Medicine: Selected Papers of Ludwig Edelstein*, ed. Owsei Temkin and C. Lilian Temkin (Baltimore: The Johns Hopkins University Press, 1967).

Oath[14] characterizes medical practitioners as a group of committed men (women were excluded from medicine in Greek society) set apart from and above others in society. Ludwig Edelstein's scholarly studies of the Oath and other Hippocratic writings have shown that this and other peculiar features of the Oath—e.g., its prohibitions against surgery, against the pharmacological inducement of abortion, and against the giving of "deadly drugs"—have their roots in the ancient Greek religious sect known as Pythagoreanism.[15] Influence from the main lines of Greek philosophical ethics seems absent, and the Oath fails to address what we would today consider fundamental ethical issues in the patient-physician relationship. Veracity and informed consent, for example, are nowhere mentioned, and most of the subjects addressed in contemporary medical ethics are not given even passing notice.

Because of its sources in the religious traditions of Pythagoreanism and its lack of a philosophical justification, the Hippocratic Oath is clearly not a philosophical document. Nonetheless, the Oath sets out some of the basic features of the beneficence model. Like oaths in general it is a solemn promise witnessed by others (in the case of ancient Greek physicians, first by a portion and then by the full panoply of the Greek gods and goddesses). By taking the Oath, one becomes committed to a distinctive moral goal or purpose of medicine as the basis of one's medical practice. Unlike descriptive or declarative statements that merely assert something, swearing an oath is a performative utterance: By subscribing to it, one is committed to live in accordance with that purpose and its implications for professional practice. The preprofessional person is transformed into the professional at least in part by the commitment ritualized in the taking of an oath. An oath, of course, is ceremonial by comparison to the commitment, which has been in formation as the young apprentice grows into the profession—i.e., is trained professionally and comes to understand and live by the obligations and virtues established in the profession.

The moral purpose of medicine appears in a central passage from the Oath: "I will apply dietetic measures to the benefit of the sick according to my ability and judgment; I will keep them from harm and injustice."[16] This statement acknowledges the physician's special knowledge and skills and his or her commitment to principles requiring the use of those skills in order to benefit patients. This, according to the Oath, is the proper moral end of medicine, and commitment to that end makes one a physician.

By itself the Hippocratic Oath is a bare skeleton of the beneficence model of moral responsibility; it sheds scant light on the concepts that de-

[14]See "Oath of Hippocrates," in Ludwig Edelstein, "The Hippocratic Oath: Text, Translation, and Interpretation," *Bulletin of the History of Medicine,* Supplement 1 (Baltimore: The Johns Hopkins University Press, 1943), p. 3.

[15]See Edelstein, *Ancient Medicine,* passim.

[16]"Oath of Hippocrates," p. 3.

fine what it means to "benefit the sick," while avoiding "harm and injustice." We must turn to other portions of the Hippocratic writings for a fuller account of the perspective from which acting in the patient's best interests is to be understood. Consider the following passage from *The Art:* "I will define what I conceive medicine to be. In general terms, it is to do away with the sufferings of the sick, to lessen the violence of their diseases, and to refuse to treat those who are overmastered by their diseases, realizing that in such cases medicine is powerless."[17]

Medicine is here conceived to have limited purposes. Its purpose is not, for example, to preserve life above all else—a distinctly modern notion.[18] Medical interventions to limit pain and suffering or to attempt curative therapy must hold out some reasonable prospect for success. This view of medicine keenly appreciates the discipline's limits. It also provides the context for the later remark in the *Epidemics:* "Declare the past, diagnose the present, foretell the future; practice these acts. As to disease, make a habit of two things—*to help, or at least to do no harm.*"[19] This text does *not* say "first (or 'above all') do no harm" (*primum non nocere,* to use a later Latin formulation).

The basic roles and concepts that give substance to the principle of beneficence in medicine are as follows: The positive benefit the physician is obligated to seek is the cure of disease and injury if there is a reasonable hope of cure; the harms to be avoided, prevented, or removed are the pain and suffering of injury and disease. In addition, the physician is enjoined from *doing* harm. This consideration, too, must be included in the beneficence model because physician interventions themselves can inflict unnecessary pain and suffering on patients. The Hippocratic texts hold that inflicting pain and suffering is permissible in those cases in which the physician is attempting to reverse a threat to health—e.g., administering an emetic[20] after the accidental ingestion of a poison. Inflicting such pain and suffering on a patient in order to eliminate a deadly substance from the body is justified because the patient is on balance benefited. When the patient cannot be benefited by further intervention, the inflicted pain and suffering is unnecessary and to be avoided. Thus, in its first formulation in Western medical ethics, the beneficence model of moral responsibility adapts the principle of beneficence to patient care by providing a medically oriented account of how to balance goods over harms.

A number of elements of the beneficence model emerge from ancient Greek medical ethics. First, the model builds its account of the moral re-

---

[17]Hippocrates, "The Art," in *Hippocrates,* trans. Jones, Vol. II, p. 193.

[18]Darrel Amundsen, "The Physician's Obligation to Prolong Life: A Medical Duty without Classical Roots," *Hastings Center Report* 8 (August 1978): 23–30.

[19]Hippocrates, "Epidemics," in *Hippocrates,* trans. Jones, Vol. I, p. 165 (emphasis added).

[20]An emetic is a substance that induces vomiting.

sponsibilities of the physician in terms of the moral purpose or end of medicine: promoting the patient's best interests as understood from medicine's perspective. Second, on this basis, it provides meanings for the key concepts in the principle of beneficence—"good" and "harm"—that are specific to medicine. In this way, the abstract principle of beneficence is adapted to the medical context. Third, it employs this principle to show that the primary, though prima facie, obligation of the physician is to benefit the patient, with prevention of unnecessary harm serving as the limiting condition.

We can now see how the beneficence model provides some distinctive direction as to how Dr. Cox might respond to Ms. Monroe's request for sterilization. The beneficence model directs Dr. Cox to consider whether sterilization is in Ms. Monroe's best interests, as those interests are understood from the objective perspective of medicine. If one assumes the Hippocratic elements of the beneficence model, it would seem that sterilization would not promote Ms. Monroe's best interests because, from the perspective of conventional medical practice, a greater balance of good over harm would not be achieved for Ms. Monroe by performing the sterilization. She does not face any significant risks to her physiological well-being by continued use of birth control pills. Indeed, she may receive significant benefits from doing so. Nor does she face significant risk to her mental well-being. While she might be frustrated by a refusal to perform the sterilization, there is no reason to suppose that her response would create more serious psychological problems. But performing the sterilization involves risks. From the perspective of medicine, these risks are not outweighed by significant benefits for the patient. Therefore, performing the sterilization would be inconsistent with the demands of the beneficence model: The procedure would not "keep her from harm."

Modern Sources of the Model

The roots of Hippocratic medical ethics, as noted above, were partially religious in character. Religious influences persisted through the many centuries that followed the early Hippocratic physicians, as did the central theme of the beneficence model: the physician's obligation to benefit patients.[21] In the modern era, religious influences on medical ethics began to be supplanted by secular influences, including philosophy. In this period, especially in the eighteenth century, the philosophical enterprise of medical ethics has its firmest roots. In both Great Britain and the United States, several influential works on medical ethics by physicians drew on philo-

---

[21]Darrel Amundsen, "Medical Ethics, History of: Medieval Europe: Fourth to Sixteenth Century," in *Encyclopedia of Bioethics*, ed. Warren T. Reich (New York: The Free Press, 1978), pp. 938–51.

sophical sources.[22] These works addressed such topics as truthfulness to the seriously ill and dying, confidentiality, and the obligation not to abandon the dying patient—all pertinent topics then, as now.

Among the most important figures in this significant historical transition was Dr. John Gregory, Professor of the Practice of Physic at Edinburgh— one of the world's great medical schools in the eighteenth century. His *Lectures on the Duties and Qualifications of a Physician* (1772)[23] was first published by his students. He then published his own version, which was issued in many editions in Great Britain, America, and the European continent, and was widely influential on medical ethics on both sides of the Atlantic well into the nineteenth century.[24] For example, Gregory's influence was felt in the United States in the first decades of the nineteenth century in the efforts of various state medical societies to formulate codes of professional ethics. Gregory was also active in the intellectual circles of his day, especially "philosophical societies" whose members included individuals learned in medicine, science, and moral philosophy. It was through such activities that Gregory came into contact with the work of leading moral philosophers of his day.[25]

Gregory begins his treatise on medical ethics with a definition of medicine that incorporates a clear expression of its moral purpose: "the art of preserving health, of prolonging life, and of curing diseases."[26] These give substance to the patient's best interests, as medicine conceives them. Like the Hippocratic writings, Gregory's *Lectures* holds that medicine has an intrinsic moral purpose. The physician is not an individual whose interests and values are simply supplemented by additional responsibilities to patients. The physician's moral role is itself understood in terms of beneficence. Gregory goes on to utilize a major philosophical concept in eighteenth-century British moral philosophy, the concept of sympathy, to build the bridge from acting in the patient's best interests to specific obligations and virtues.

Although it is not precisely known which of his contemporaries' works were the source of Gregory's use of the concept of sympathy, we shall expli-

---

[22]For an overview of this period, see section on "Medical Ethics, History of: Modern Period: Seventeenth to Nineteenth Century," articles by L. B. McCullough, A. R. Jonsen, C. R. Burns, G. B. Risse, D. B. Weiner, and M. J. Peterson, in *Encyclopedia of Bioethics*, pp. 951–75. See also Darrel W. Amundsen and Gary Ferngren, "Philanthropy in Medicine: Some Historical Perspectives," in *Beneficence and Health Care*, ed. Earl Shelp, pp. 1–32.

[23]John Gregory, *Lectures on the Duties and Qualifications of a Physician* (London: W. Strahan, 1772). Quoted passages taken from 1817 edition published by M. Carey & Son of Philadelphia.

[24]Chester Burns, "Reciprocity in Anglo-American Medical Ethics, 1765–1865," in *Proceedings of the XXIII International Congress of the History of Medicine* (London, 1974), pp. 813–19.

[25]See Ernest Campbell Mossner, *The Life of David Hume*. 2d ed. (Oxford: Clarendon Press, 1980), pp. 273, 580–81.

[26]John Gregory, *Lectures on the Duties and Qualifications of a Physician*, p. 6.

cate this concept along the lines proposed by David Hume. (Gregory was well aware of Hume's work, even if he was not always in sympathy with it.) According to Hume, moral judgments are not ultimately based in reason, but rather in the natural human disposition of sympathy. Sympathy allows one to put oneself in another's place so as to feel what the other is feeling and thus become "sympathetic" with the other's circumstance. "Were I present at any of the more terrible operations of surgery," writes Hume, "the preparation of the instruments, the laying of the bandages in order, the heating of the irons, with all the signs of anxiety and concern in the patient and assistants, would have a great effect upon my mind, and excite the strongest sentiments of pity and terror."[27] Such pain and suffering of another is unpleasant to us, Hume argues, and we sense their feelings, thus giving rise to sympathy. This is what often moves physicians to act in the best interests of their patients, Hume would conclude.

Gregory's extensive use of sympathy exhibits important similarities to Hume's. For example, through the medium of sympathy the physician appreciates the importance of the duty to maintain confidentiality. The physician realizes "how much the character of individuals, and the credit of families, may sometimes depend on the discretion, secrecy, and honour of the physician."[28] Gregory also recognizes the prima facie character of the physician's obligations in his account of the duties and virtues of truthfulness, for example. (We examine this topic at greater length in the next chapter.)

> A physician is often at a loss when speaking to his patients of their real situation when it is dangerous. A deviation from truth is sometimes in this case both justifiable and necessary. It often happens that a person is extremely ill; but yet may recover, if he be not informed of his danger. It sometimes happens, on the other hand, that a man is seized with a dangerous illness, who has made no settlement of his affairs: and yet perhaps the future happiness of his family may depend on his making such a settlement. In this and other similar cases, it may be proper for a physician, in the most prudent and gentle manner, to give a hint to the patient of his real danger, and even solicit him to set about this necessary duty.[29]

Here sympathy is applied to help the physician appreciate the tragic consequences that might befall the patient's family should he die without having prepared his estate. The result of applying the principle of beneficence is that the physician has a prima facie obligation to be truthful to the dying.

In his medical ethics, Gregory also places considerable emphasis on the virtues, which are underemphasized in the Hippocratic writings. In particular, he notes that in all cases of conflict between the physician's personal

---

[27]David Hume, *A Treatise of Human Nature*, ed. L. A. Selby-Bigge, 2d ed. rev. P. H. Nidditch (Oxford: Oxford University Press, 1978), Book III, p. 576.

[28]John Gregory, *Lectures on the Duties and Qualifications of a Physician*, pp. 29–30.

[29]Ibid., 36.

interests and his or her obligations to patients, virtue requires that the latter come first. Being honest with seriously ill patients, as every physician has experienced, is often a difficult matter, and Gregory is quick to agree. Nevertheless, he holds that the obligation to benefit patients outweighs the physician's personal discomfort in carrying out the moral responsibility to tell a patient that death is imminent.

> To a man of a compassionate and feeling heart, this [honest disclosure] is one of the most disagreeable duties in the profession: but it is indispensible. The manner of doing it, requires equal prudence and humanity. What should reconcile him the more easily to this painful office, is the reflection that, if the patient should recover, it will prove a joyful disappointment to his friends; and if he die, it makes the shock more gentle.[30]

This same line of reasoning also applies to interprofessional conflict that distracts attention from the care of patients, again clearly reflecting the main lines of the beneficence model: "There are often unhappy jealousies and animosities among those of the profession, by which their patients may suffer . . . . Physicians . . . should divest themselves of all particularities, and think of nothing but what will most effectively contribute to the relief of those under their care."[31]

A complete account of the moral responsibilities of physicians thus requires, for Gregory, reference to those virtues that keep the physician's attention fixed on his or her obligations to patients and their best interests, rather than on the physician's personal interests. In the case of truth-telling, Gregory emphasizes the virtues of prudence and humanity. The first is required so that the physician is aware of the harm that untimely revelations might cause, while the second reminds the physician of the importance of the style employed in conveying dismaying or tragic information to the patient. More generally, Gregory calls for those virtues that enable the physician to be a person "who feels the misfortunes of . . . fellow creatures."[32] At the same time, the physician should not be overly sympathetic with the patient, for this invites unsteadiness and misjudgment. On his list of the virtues are not only patience, good nature, generosity, and compassion, but steadiness and vigor as well.[33]

Gregory's medical ethics provides us with all the elements of the beneficence model. He first defines the moral end or purpose of medicine and the way the principle of beneficence is adapted to clinical practice through the medium of sympathy. He delineates obligations generated by this principle, such as confidentiality and truth-telling to the terminally ill. Finally,

---

[30]Ibid., 37.
[31]Ibid., 38.
[32]Ibid., 12.
[33]Ibid., 12–13.

he insists on the importance of virtues that are essential to the routine and humane fulfillment of the physician's obligations. Gregory and many others in the history of medicine reveal how physicians are morally obligated to benefit patients because of a role they have voluntarily assumed. Obligations and virtues of beneficence are built into the very understanding of the relationship between patients and physicians. The institution of medicine itself leads to the Hippocratic Oath, through which the physician pledges to come "for the benefit of the sick." Thus, the physician on duty in an emergency room is obligated by his or her role to attend to an injured, delirious, uncooperative patient, sometimes at considerable personal risk. This is the contemporary legacy in medicine of such writings as those of Gregory and the Hippocratic physicians, because this conduct puts the patient's best interest first and fulfills the physician's obligations to the patient.

In the history of medicine, the physician has primarily functioned in care-giving and comforting roles, with beneficence serving as the moral foundation of these roles. As medical science exploded in the twentieth century, medicine was transformed into a more scientific and technical enterprise. It might be argued that this change has transformed the physician's role, stripping it of its moral core and making it a *sheerly* technical enterprise. However, this hypothesis is misleading. Beneficent intervention remains, as ever, the moral foundation of the physician's role, a role powerfully augmented by medical science and technology. These remarkable new capacities created some moral problems in medicine, especially problems concerning the physician's authority, but they did not destroy medicine's tradition of beneficence. In chapters three through five we encounter this legacy of the past as the living reality of the beneficence model in contemporary medicine.

Uses and Abuses of the Model

Unlike the compassionate approach *intrinsic* to the beneficence model, this same model is occasionally applied in quite uncompromising ways that are in unnecessary opposition to the autonomy model. For example, in a recent discussion of the case of a Jehovah's Witness who experienced heavy bleeding following the delivery of her third child (because of a rupture of her uterus), Dr. John Jewett pointedly expressed his view of the moral status of her refusal of a blood transfusion and eventual death from total exsanguination: "The record thereafter is one of unremitting effort frustrated by intransigent adherence to a dogma inimical to life. The patient, her husband, and above all, the adviser, must accept responsibility for this needless death."[34] Several letters appeared in response to Dr. Jewett's case

[34]John Figgis Jewett, "Report from the Committee on Maternal Welfare: Total Exsanguination," *New England Journal of Medicine* 305 (12 November 1981): 1218.

report. One physician, Dr. Harold Hanzlik, reported on a similar case, but one in which the patient lived "with a markedly diminished intellectual capacity from prolonged cerebral hypoxia and with the loss of several fingers and toes from gangrene,"[35] following a three-month hospital course. Dr. Hanzlik's remarks are equally uncompromising in appealing to the beneficence model: "Is there any legal mechanism—or can there ever be—for overriding a cult that forbids medical experts to act?"[36]

In his reply to the letters, Dr. Jewett speaks on behalf of the Committee on Maternal Welfare of the Massachusetts Medical Society, of which he is Chair. "The committee," he declares, "considers itself incompetent to compare the relative values of physical and eternal life, but can reaffirm without equivocation that the premature transition from one to the other was absolutely unnecessary."[37] Medicine includes as one of its core values the prolongation of life by preventing premature death, which Dr. Jewett believes was his patient's fate. While treatment was not forced on this patient, Dr. Jewitt seems of the view, fashioned from the beneficence model, that it was morally irresponsible of the patient to have refused treatment and that physicians should not be shackled by law or ethics from acting in their patients' best interests even in the face of an autonomous refusal. This is an injudicious interpretation of the demands of the beneficence model, and we shall ultimately reject it because of its implications for autonomous choice by patients.

In an article published at the same time as Dr. Jewett's, Dr. J. Lowell Dixon argued for a more balanced perspective on the demands of what we have termed the beneficence model.[38] He recognizes that "caring for Jehovah's Witnesses might seem to pose a dilemma for the physician dedicated to preserving life and health by employing all the techniques at his disposal."[39] Dr. Dixon argues that some physicians have viewed Jehovah's Witness patients as challenges rather than problems and have been able to devise special treatment modalities, including surgery, that are consistent with the moral demands of Witnesses' religious faith. Dr. Dixon concludes that "These physicians are at the same time providing care that is best for the patient's total good."[40] It is clearly a mistake to interpret the benefi-

[35]Harold Hanzlik, "Total Exsanguination After Refusal of Blood Transfusions" (Letter), *New England Journal of Medicine* 306 (4 March 1982): 544.

[36]Ibid. Dr. Jewett does not *always* suggest that the beneficence model trumps the autonomy model. Indeed, he suggests the reverse weighting in "Pulmonary Hypertension and Pre-Eclampsia," *New England Journal of Medicine* 301 (8 November 1979): 1063–64.

[37]John Figgis Jewett, "Total Exsanguination After Refusal of Blood Transfusions" (Letter), *New England Journal of Medicine* 306 (4 March 1982): 545.

[38]J. Lowell Dixon and M. Gene Smalley, "Jehovah's Witnesses: The Surgical/Ethical Challenge," *Journal of the American Medical Association* 246 (27 November 1981): 2471–72.

[39]Ibid. 2472.

[40]Ibid.

cence model as the justification for an imperious attitude, such as that apparently adopted by Dr. Jewett, rather than as a posture of discretion and compromise that implements the demands of the beneficence model in a more humane fashion, such as that exhibited by Dr. Dixon.

Just as a commitment to the well-being of Jehovah's Witness patients has led to recent innovations in their medical care, so too a general commitment to the beneficence model has served as a profound moral motivation for the important medical practices of caring, sacrifice, compassion, sympathy, and determination to develop, test, or apply diagnostic and treatment modalities. This tradition has sometimes even achieved heroic proportions, as in the case of the physicians who remained in East Coast cities during the Yellow Fever epidemics of the eighteenth century, or in the case of the physicians who went into Hiroshima and Nagasaki after the explosion of atomic bombs in 1945. But even in routine practice, this tradition has been partially responsible for the deeply respected status medicine occupies as a profession. The fact that some physicians sometimes carry it to disturbing extremes provides no cause for neglecting its lustrous past or its continuing power as a model of behavior.

The Elements of the Model

While historical sources and contemporary examples are crucial for our attempt to understand the beneficence model, they must be supplemented by the critical and constructive analysis that philosophical reasoning provides. This model is built on a conception of goods and harms that underlie applications of the principle of beneficence in the model, and our construction of the model must begin with these goods and harms as medicine understands them. We believe that the following list expresses what medicine is to seek and avoid.[41]

Goods	Harms
Health	Illness
Prevention, elimination, or control of disease (morbidity) and injury	Disease (morbidity) and injury
Relief from unnecessary pain and suffering	Unnecessary pain and suffering
Amelioration of handicapping conditions	Handicapping conditions
Prolonged life	Premature death

[41]We draw this list of medical goods and harms from both historical and contemporary sources. See also Eric Cassell, "The Nature of Suffering and the Goals of Medicine," *New England Journal of Medicine* 306 (18 March 1982): 639. This list of goods and harms does not differ significantly from that offered by, for example, Albert R. Jonsen et al. in *Clinical Ethics*, pp. 13–14. We view educating and counseling patients (their #5) as a *means* to securing the goods on their list.

The goods and harms accepted by the beneficence model are rarely discussed in modern medicine as *values,* perhaps because they are such deeply embedded presuppositions in clinical practice and training. Increasingly, however, physicians are becoming aware of how these basic values, and many judgments derived from them, shape clinical decisionmaking. Even in highly quantified clinical decisionmaking, value judgments may be at work. Subtle tradeoffs, for example, between different levels of medically induced (iatrogenic) morbidity may be under constant evaluation.[42] Some specific examples will illustrate how such reasoning plays a role in medicine.

Consider the prophylactic use of drugs to reduce the risk of coronary and cerebrovascular disease in individuals at risk for such disease. Dr. Michael Oliver has argued that for patients who are otherwise healthy, a balance must be struck between maintaining health and risking illness caused by the use of these drugs. He calls for a change in current practice by limiting the use of prophylactic treatment to only those cases where there is good evidence, and not mere supposition, to believe that the benefits outweigh the risks.[43]

Drs. James Reuler and Donald Girard have identified how considerations about pain and its relief should figure in the primary physician's management of elderly patients with cancer.[44] They first distinguish benign forms of chronic pain in patients without cancer and argue that addicting drugs, with the morbidity and suffering they cause, should not be used for such pain. The presence of cancer in an elderly patient, however, leads them to change their balancing of these goods and harms. In these cases, the physician should be concerned not only about the relief of pain but about the patient's anxiety that medication will not be administered unless or until the pain renews its onslaught. Such anxiety can be a significant form of suffering for such patients. Hence, they argue that pain medications, including those with addictive potential, should be administered to cancer patients as required.

Dr. Wilton Bunch argues that protocols for the treatment of osteochondroses will differ because of value judgments implicit in each treatment.[45] These value judgments involve, he claims, a balancing between the good of ameliorating handicapping conditions and avoiding in-

---

[42]Allan S. Brett, "Hidden Ethical Issues in Clinical Decision Analysis," *New England Journal of Medicine* 305 (5 November 1981): 1150–52.

[43]Michael F. Oliver, "Risks of Correcting the Risks of Coronary Disease and Stroke with Drugs," *New England Journal of Medicine* 306 (4 February 1982): 297–98.

[44]James B. Reuler and Donald E. Girard, "The Primary Care Physician's Role in Cancer Management," *Geriatrics* 36 (November 1981): 41–50.

[45]Wilton Bunch, "Decision Analysis of Treatment Choices in the Osteochondroses," *Clinical Orthopedics* 158 (July–August 1981): 91–98. Osteochondrosis is a degenerative disease of the bone.

creased morbidity. In addressing the surgical management of deformities of the lower extremities of patients with cerebral palsy, Dr. Robert Samilson argues that the general goal of such surgical treatment is increased function.[46] At the same time, the burdens of surgery should not be imposed in every case of the loss of function in the lower extremities. Surgery is acceptable only when the handicap to be corrected or ameliorated promotes the patient's overall well-being, e.g., enabling the patient to sit erect or to flex the knee.

Finally, Dr. Paul Brown identifies similar judgments that must be made in cases of orthopedic surgery where the alternatives are surgical amputation involving the upper extremities and an attempt to reattach, for example, a severed finger. In language remarkably similar to Dr. Gregory's, Dr. Brown develops the duties and virtues that characterize the beneficence model.[47] After a review of the literature, together with a discussion of clinical experience, Dr. Brown concludes that the relevant goods and harms are not simply those of having or not having one's finger remain part of one's body. The good of the reattachment of one's finger must be weighed against the possibility that it may be nonfunctional or only partly functional or even aesthetically displeasing to the patient. In some cases, he concludes, amputation may be more consistent with the patient's best interests than reattachment.

As these examples indicate, in applications of the principle of beneficence in medicine, goods of medical intervention must constantly be weighed against risks of harms presented by disease and handicaps, as well as by the medical interventions themselves. Beneficence includes the obligation to balance benefits against harms, benefits against alternative benefits, and harms against alternative harms. It also requires that the physician maintain the professional skills required to properly weigh and balance the alternatives. (Here, "Know your business" becomes a moral imperative ingredient in the model itself.) If this balancing leads a physician to conceive his or her obligations to patients differently from patients' assessments, the beneficence model simply dictates that the physician act in accordance with the ends of medicine. Therefore, the physician cannot kill, assist suicide, administer drugs with no hope of a medically indicated effect, and the like. However, the model has no power to show that the physician's medical judgment must *always* override the patient's. The model simply frames the physician's obligations in terms of medically specific ways of providing benefits and avoiding harms.

The elements of the beneficence model build on each other to provide an integrated account of the moral dimensions of the physician's role—its

[46]Robert L. Samilson, "Current Concepts of Surgical Management of Deformities of the Lower Extremities in Cerebral Palsy," *Clinical Orthopedics* 158 (July–August 1981): 99–107.

[47]Paul W. Brown, "The Rational Selection of Treatment for Upper Extremity Amputations," *Orthopedic Clinics of North America* 12 (October 1981): 843–48.

moral end, its moral principle, its moral obligations, and its moral virtues. In schematic form, these elements are as follows:

1. *The Moral End of Medicine:* The end of medicine is the promotion of the patient's best interest, as understood from the perspective of medicine.
2. *Basic Moral Principle:* The principle of beneficence is the sole fundamental principle. It requires the physician to promote goods for patients, as medicine sees those goods, and to avoid harms, as medicine sees those harms.
3. *Derivative Moral Obligations:* From the principle of beneficence the physician's role-related obligations are derived: honest communication, confidentiality, fidelity, and the like.
4. *Derivative Moral Virtues:* From the principle of beneficence the physician's role-related virtues are also derived: truthfulness, trustworthiness, faithfulness, and the like.

Case Applications

We are now in a position to see in greater detail how the beneficence model would help Dr. Cox address the moral problem confronting her. Among the possible *goods* for Ms. Monroe are not having children, pursuing her career goals, controlling her reproductive capacity, avoiding the risks of alternative reversible means of birth control (particularly the IUD), avoiding the long-term risks (beyond age 35) of the use of the birth control pill, and benefiting from disease-preventing aspects of long-term use of the birth control pill. Among the possible *harms* for Ms. Monroe are the disruptions to her career caused by becoming pregnant or becoming a parent, the disappointment at never having children, the risks of laparoscopy, the long-term risks of tubal ligation, and the long-term risks of using the birth control pill. Which among these harms and goods should be given the greatest weight in Dr. Cox's determination of her obligations to Ms. Monroe?

The beneficence model could be invoked to answer this question in several steps. Because it takes *medicine's* perspective on a patient's best interests, the model first clarifies which among the many possible general goods and harms for Ms. Monroe count as goods and harms in that perspective. The following list defines what medicine takes to be Ms. Monroe's best interests:

Goods	Harms
Avoiding the medical complications of alternative reversible methods of birth control	Medical complications of laparoscopy
Avoiding the long-term medical complications of the birth control pill	Long-term medical complications of the birth control pill
Disease-preventing aspects of long-term use of the birth control pill	Long-term medical complications of tubal ligation

Other possible goods and harms listed earlier are undoubtedly of overriding concern to Ms. Monroe, but from the perspective of the beneficence model these goals or desires on the patient's part are not primary, because they do not involve the patient's health. (Under the autonomy model, we shall see that those goals do become primary.) Dr. Cox must determine whether sterilization or continuing on the birth control pill satisfies the criterion of the patient's medical best interests. The latter course poses acceptable risks (until at least the age of 35) and may even have some medical benefits for patients like Ms. Monroe. The former course, however, carries with it the risks of a surgical procedure and the long-term risks of sterilization. It does not bring a greater balance of benefit over harm, from medicine's perspective. Instead, the balance of good over harm seems clearly to favor Ms. Monroe's continued use of the birth control pill. This is where the "weight of morality" rests if one takes the perspective of the beneficence model; and thus Dr. Cox should not perform the sterilization if the criteria in this model are taken to be solely decisive.

If a declaration to this effect were the sole directive of the beneficence model, it would be cold and harsh indeed, directing Dr. Cox simply to reply "No" to Ms. Monroe's request, without further explanation. Gregory's emphasis on virtue—which we take to be central to the model—contrasts noticeably. He would direct Dr. Cox to communicate in a sympathetic and compassionate way the reasons why performing the sterilization is inconsistent with the moral demands of the beneficence model. Dr. Cox has already laid the groundwork for this approach by sharing her own life experience with Ms. Monroe. This information should help her explore her motivations for having the sterilization performed.

We can easily imagine Ms. Monroe at this point asking Dr. Cox for a referral. How might Dr. Cox respond to such a request while remaining faithful to the beneficence model? At a minimum, Dr. Cox should not take offense at Ms. Monroe's request and should reject any feeling of interprofessional rivalry, as Dr. Gregory cautioned. Dr. Cox should explain how she has attempted to assess goods and harms objectively for Ms. Monroe, and she might mention that it is therefore likely that another physician will agree that the sterilization should not be performed. Nonetheless, Dr. Cox might acknowledge that because Ms. Monroe may be at risk for complications from long-term use of the birth control pill, another physician might arrive at a different assessment. Certainly Dr. Cox should not hesitate to refer Ms. Monroe merely because she takes the perspective of the beneficence model, for that model will not sustain the conclusion that referral is inappropriate.

More importantly, the beneficence model is not the only possible source a physician might tap in order to determine the patient's best interest. The *patient's* perspective might be taken as having equal, or even decisive weight. We turn now to the model of the moral responsibility of physicians based in the perspective of autonomy.

THE AUTONOMY MODEL

In contrast to the beneficence model, the autonomy model takes the *values and beliefs of the patient* to be the primary moral consideration in determining the physician's moral responsibilities in patient care: If the patient's values directly conflict with medicine's values, the fundamental responsibility of physicians is to respect and to facilitate a patient's self-determination in making decisions about his or her medical fate. The obligations and virtues of the physician thus flow from the principle of respect for autonomy. This model is not without support in the history of medical ethics, but has its major sources in the histories of law and philosophy.

Legal Sources of the Model

A key feature of the principle of respect for autonomy has been developed in legal contexts, where "self-determination" has a venerable history and is taken to be synonymous with what we are calling autonomy—that is, the ability to understand one's situation and pursue personal goals free of governing constraints. The principle of self-determination means that one has sovereignty over one's life—a sovereignty that protects privacy as well as rights to control what happens to one's person and property. In its original development in the law, the intrinsic worth of the individual, including the right to personal sovereignty, was advanced primarily as a check or limit on the authority of the state or another person. For example, the Bill of Rights and the "due process" amendments to the United States Constitution were so fashioned. The central theme is that a person's sovereignty limits the sphere into which others may legitimately intrude.

Individual sovereignty needs protection for two reasons. First, there is a danger of imbalance in power between the individual and the state (or other parties) in favor of the latter. Individual rights provide a corrective to this imbalance by insuring that individuals as individuals will be given due consideration and respect. Second, conflicts arise between an individual's perception of his or her best interests and another's perception of those interests. Rights of individual sovereignty protect an individual's freedom to choose his or her best interests. The legal principle of respect for self-determination is applied to questions concerning the physician's responsibility because patients and physicians are unequal in their possession of information and their power to control the circumstances under which they meet. Typically, one party is fit and medically knowledgeable, the other sick and medically ignorant.[48] Legal rights are a way of limiting the physi-

---

[48]Drummond Rennie, "Informed Consent by 'Well-Nigh Abject' Adults," *New England Journal of Medicine* 302 (17 April 1980): 917.

cian's power and of protecting the patient from unwarranted intrusions—such as surgery without consent, involuntary commitment to a mental institution, and public disclosure of information contained in hospital records.

Conflicts also arise between medicine's understanding of a patient's best interests and the patient's understanding of those interests. This conflict occurs in the case that opens this chapter. Ms. Monroe views sterilization as a means of securing her goals of controlling conception and not having children, and these goods and harms—not the goods and harms of the beneficence model—define her best interests. A physician, we saw, may view this patient's best interests in quite another way by following the beneficence model. Thus, the law dictates that the physician who performs an invasive procedure without the patient's permission may be found guilty of a *battery,* though usually only *negligence* is charged. The underlying rationale behind the battery theory of liability for failure to obtain the patient's agreement has been closely linked in law to autonomy. This rationale burst on the scene in a crucial 1914 case and has since been widely offered as the basic right underlying the legal doctrine of informed consent (which we explore in chapter three): "Every human being of adult years and sound mind has a right to determine what shall be done with his own body; and a surgeon who performs an operation without his patient's consent commits an assault."[49]

This right is an autonomy right. The language in which the law has expressed it is quite striking. Among the most important formulations is the following from a 1960 landmark case, *Natanson v. Kline:* "A doctor might well believe that an operation or form of treatment is desirable or necessary but the law does not permit him to substitute his own judgment for that of the patient by any form of artifice or deception."[50] In a later case, Warren Burger, who later became Chief Justice of the United States Supreme Court, amplified the legal concept of self-determination, with a reflection on the character of the reasons or values of a patient that are meant to be protected. He argued that nothing in the right to be left alone means that an individual possesses these rights only regarding sensible beliefs, reasonable emotions, and the like. Hence many eccentric and even absurd ideas may validly form the basis of a patient's autonomous choices.[51] The physician thus is not free to transfuse a Jehovah's Witness who autonomously refuses life-saving blood products, even if, as in the case discussed in Dr. Jewett's report, the physican values prolonged life and feels obligated to avoid premature death in the best interests of the patient.

[49]*Schloendorff v. Society of New York Hospitals,* 211 N.Y. 125, p. 127; 105 N. E. 92 (1914). See chapter five, pp. 63–64.

[50]*Natanson v. Kline.* 186 Kan. 393. 350 P.2d 1093 (1969). 187 Kan. 186, 354 P.2d 670 (1960). See chapter three, p. 65.

[51]*Application of the President and Directors of Georgetown College, Inc.,* 331 F.2d 1010 (D.C. Cir. 1964). Certiorari denied, 337 U.S. 978 (1964).

The relationship between patients and physicians is seen by the law in contractual and fiduciary terms. The implications for the responsibilities of the physician are clear and forceful. The physician is not to assume that, simply because an individual is under the physician's care, the physician is therefore free (as the *fiduciary*) to pursue the best interests of the patient as medicine might conceive them. To do so would be to deny the "equal standing" ingredient in the contractual dimension of the patient-physician relationship. The physician's responsibility cannot be sharply divorced from the patient's self-determined choices and decisions, including best interests as defined by the patient. Thus, based on this model alone, Dr. Cox should perform the sterilization Ms. Monroe has requested.

Philosophical Sources of the Model

Like the Hippocratic Oath, the word "autonomy" is a legacy from ancient Greece. The Greek *autos* (self) and *nomos* (rule or law) first combined to refer to self-governance in the Greek city-state. The most general idea of personal autonomy in moral philosophy is still self-governance: forming one's own self by adequate knowledge and understanding, free from controlling interferences by others or by personal limitations. The general idea of autonomy is linked in philosophical literature to several allied concepts, such as the freedom to choose, the creation of a personal moral position, and accepting responsibility for one's actions. There is near uniform agreement in this literature that a person lacking critical internal capacities for self-rule—and not mere freedom from external controls or constraints—lacks something integral to self-governance. Thus the autonomous person is both free of external control and in control of his or her affairs. One is autonomous in this sense only if one is capable of controlled deliberation and free action.

While a more precise analysis of autonomy remains a matter of philosophical controversy, we define an autonomous decision as follows: A person's decision is autonomous if it derives from the person's own values and beliefs, is based on adequate information and understanding, and is not determined by internal or external constraints that compel the decision. A person's autonomy is reduced if some of these conditions are unsatisfied or only weakly satisfied. We shall provide further analysis of this definition both in chapter five, where the subject of reduced autonomy is related to that of diminished competence, and in chapter three, where the nature of decisionmaking by patients is examined.

Respect for autonomy in this context suggests a morally appropriate *attitude*, and we shall therefore sometimes speak of virtues of respectfulness. More commonly, however, the focus will be on the obligations generated by the autonomous patient's *right* to be respected and to take actions based on personal beliefs and values. From this position, the burden of proof rests on one who would intervene by restricting or preventing a person's exercise of an autonomy right. Respect for autonomy thus implies noninterference with that person's beliefs, values, and rights, as well as noninterference with and acceptance of choices that express them.

A *principle* of respect for autonomy requires that persons be enabled to order their values and beliefs and to choose and act free from the controlling interventions of others. Even if risk that to others may appear foolhardy is involved, this principle demands noninterference and respect as the proper responses to the autonomous choices of persons. For example, autonomous, informed patients have the right to decide that medical intervention to prevent death is unacceptable; these patients have the right to refuse further treatment, even in the face of certain death.[52] However, such rights do not always have overriding authority, and hence the burden of proof for an intervention can in principle be met. *How* it can be met is a central concern of chapters three through six.

The philosophical roots of this principle of respect for autonomy are not as easily traceable to ancient Greece as are the Hippocratic roots of the beneficence model. Indeed, their most prominent formulations are found in the philosophical ethics of the seventeenth and eighteenth centuries. In particular, the work of the British philosopher John Locke[53] and the German philosopher Immanuel Kant[54] have proven to be of monumental historical influence. Locke was concerned about the power of the state and the protection of individual rights. He delineated both a sphere of individual autonomy that any morally just state must respect and a doctrine of basic entitlements to noninterference that every individual possesses prior to the formation of a political order. There are four such rights in Locke's system: the rights to life, liberty, health, and possessions. The state cannot interfere with these rights without a valid authorization from the individual. Like the legal principle of respect for self-determination, Locke's rights protect against intervention without consent.

There is, however, more to the principle of respect for autonomy in the history of philosophy than Locke's orientation. Philosophers after Locke generally deemphasized the relationship between the citizen and the state. Kant's theory is especially noteworthy. He was interested in the conditions for the establishment of a moral community whose defining mark would be mutual respect. A requirement that we treat one another as free to choose is fundamental for him. We thus should not treat others as means to our

---

[52]President's Commission for the Study of Ethical Problems in Medicine and Biomedical and Behavioral Research, *Deciding to Forego Life-Sustaining Treatment* (Washington, D.C.: U.S. Government Printing Office, 1983), p. 244ff; and (for the theoretical grounding of this claim in autonomy) *Making Health Care Decisions* (Washington, D.C.: U.S. Government Printing Office, 1982), p. 44ff., esp. p. 47.

[53]John Locke, *Two Treatises of Government,* ed. Peter Laslett (Cambridge: Cambridge University Press, 1960).

[54]Immanuel Kant, *Groundwork of the Metaphysic of Morals,* trans. H. J. Paton (New York: Harper & Row, 1964).

own ends (i.e., just as we please) without their consent. To do so would involve disrespect for their autonomous determinations, and so would disrespect them as autonomous agents. Thus, in evaluating the decisions and actions of others, we have a duty to accord them the same right to their judgments that we possess, and they in turn must treat us in the same way.

Following the courses charted by Locke and Kant, subsequent moral philosophy has generally supported the following interpretation of the principle of respect for autonomy: Autonomous decisions and actions should not be constrained by others. Two observations are in order about this principle: (1) As formulated, this broad principle has no exceptions built into it that express valid conditions or interventions that allow us to limit autonomy. However, respect for autonomy is a prima facie principle, and so can be overridden by other moral principles that permit constraints on autonomy. (2) All persons who do not have informational or related mental deficiencies or some form of internal or external governing constraints on their will are autonomous and can make autonomous decisions. All persons of this description fall under the scope of this principle. However, the principle of respect for autonomy must not be interpreted as applying to all individuals. Some individuals fail to act autonomously because they are incapacitated or coerced. Someone with reduced autonomy is highly dependent on others and in at least some respect incapable of making choices based on controlled deliberations. For example, young children, drug addicts, senile individuals, and many institutionalized populations, such as the mentally retarded, may suffer from reduced autonomy. For such persons the principle of respect for autonomy may be inapplicable. As we shall see in chapter five, many patients cannot, without significant qualifications, be described as autonomous. There are also many conflicts between the principle of respect for autonomy and beneficence.

Relevance to Medical Practice

There are innumerable examples of the application of the autonomy model to patient care, both in the history of medicine and in contemporary medical literature. For example, the views of Richard Clarke Cabot on truthfulness to patients, examined in chapter one, have their roots in respect for the autonomy of the patient. Like Gregory before him, Dr. Cabot was aware of the difficulties and discomforts caused for the physician by a practice of veracity. Yet Dr. Cabot makes an explicitly Kantian argument in favor of truthfulness to patients and against lying as the basis for his injunction that physicians are obligated to practice veracity in communicating with patients.[55]

---

[55]Dr. Cabot writes the following: "Now a lie seems to me to do something like that. By undermining the confidence of man in man it does its part in making not one but every human activity impossible. If we cannot trust one another, we cannot take a step in any direction. Business, social relations, science, everything worth doing depends on mutual confidence. It is

The autonomy model has received its most persistent application in medicine in the rules governing informed consent. In a contemporary study of medical decisionmaking, Drs. Stephen Eraker and Peter Politser note a recent shift in the place that patient's values are given in medical decisions: "As medical decisions become technically more complex and are associated with greater costs to the patient, physicians have been increasingly motivated to incorporate patient preferences in these critical decisions."[56] These writers also emphasize the importance of controlling biases derived from the perspective of medicine that are common in decisionmaking: "If physicians are to better serve the patient's best interests they must understand the way patients perceive and evaluate medical risks and benefits."[57]

A recent study of laryngeal cancer also shows the import of the autonomy model. In stage T3 carcinoma of the larynx, which is restricted to the vocal cords and causes their immobility, laryngectomy (extirpation or partial excision of the larynx) causes loss of normal speech and holds out a sixty percent likelihood of survival for three years. By contrast, radiation therapy holds out a thirty to forty percent likelihood of survival for three years, but it preserves normal speech or its functional equivalent. A study by three physicians in the Department of Radiology and Radiation Therapy at the Harvard Medical School and the Department of Medicine at the Tufts School of Medicine examined which therapy autonomous patients would choose. They discovered that nineteen percent would choose radiation therapy if a forty percent likelihood of survival were projected, and that twenty-four percent would choose this course if a delayed laryngectomy were planned. These physicians argue that such quality-of-life tradeoffs are integral to the decision process for patients and therefore should be carefully explained as viable options more often than they generally are in medicine.

If medicine proceeds *exclusively* on a beneficence model, such information might never be transmitted to patients. The decision for a therapy would be made by the conventions of medical practice, and—as these investigators stress—radiation therapy is considered a "relatively unconventional treatment" in contemporary medicine. The overall conclusion they draw from their study involves a direct application of the autonomy model:

> The importance of integrating attitudes toward the length of survival and the quality of life is clear. First of all, it is known that persons have different preferences for length of survival: Some place greater value on proximate years than on distant years. . . .

---

the very air we breathe. To poison it is to do a thing far worse for society than the loss of a single life." Richard C. Cabot, "The Use of Truth and Falsehood in Medicine," *American Medicine* 5 (1903): 344–49, reprinted in Stanley Reiser et al., *Ethics in Medicine* (Cambridge: MIT Press, 1977), p. 218.

[56]Stephen Eraker and Peter Politser, "How Decisions are Reached: Physician and Patient," *Annals of Internal Medicine* 97 (1982): 262.

[57]Ibid., 267.

This study has a straightforward message: Patients' attitudes toward morbidity are important, and survival is not their only consideration. Such attitudes vary enormously from patient to patient. These results seem to preclude paternalistic decisions based on "my clinical experience with patients who have your disease." Future work to improve the methods for assessing mortality and morbidity is obviously necessary. In the meantime, this study suggests that major attempts should be made to incorporate patients' attitudes toward the quality and quantity of life into the decision-making process.[58]

The case of Ms. Monroe illustrates many of these same problems of respect for autonomy in medicine. Ms. Monroe requires the assistance of a physician to implement her decision to destroy her anatomical capacity to conceive. Based on the principle of respect for autonomy alone, Dr. Cox seems obligated to respect the decision and perhaps to perform the sterilization. After all, Ms. Monroe has given careful thought to her decision. While the risks of sterilization appear to be marginally more significant than those of continued use of the birth control pill, and while sterilization would not offer the possible benefits of long-term use of the pill, Ms. Monroe nonetheless is willing, on the basis of her values and beliefs, to accept those risks and forego those benefits in order to realize her values. Indeed, she might ask, why undergo the risks of the birth control pill? She does not intend to have children and will seek an irreversible means of fertility control anyway when the pill later becomes marginally more risky than sterilization. But is Dr. Cox obligated not only to listen and counsel carefully, but also to *act* on Ms. Monroe's request? This question raises issues not only about obligations generated by the principle of respect for autonomy but about competing obligations and also about virtues required to fulfill those obligations. We shall return to some of these issues after a brief discussion of the elements of the autonomy model.

The Elements of the Model

While historical sources and contemporary examples are crucial for our attempt to understand the autonomy model, they require critical and constructive philosophical shaping—a task to which we now turn. Like the beneficence model, the autonomy model takes its beginning in the moral injunction to promote the patient's best interests. The distinctive feature of the autonomy model is its insistence that the individual patient's perspective on and interpretation of his or her best interests is fundamental.

No independent, objective list of medical goods and harms can be developed that is comparable to the list in the beneficence model because the

---

[58]Barbara J. McNeil, Ralph Weichselbaum, and Stephen G. Pauker, "Speech and Survival: Tradeoffs Between Quality and Quantity of Life in Laryngeal Cancer," *The New England Journal of Medicine* 305 (22 October 1981): 987.

individual's perspective is vastly more individualistic than the objective medical perspective that defines goods and harms in the beneficence model. Ms. Monroe's acceptance of the marginally greater health risks of tubal ligation and rejection of the marginally greater benefits of continuing on birth control pills is but one of many idiosyncratic but nonetheless autonomous judgments by patients that deviate sharply from the risk/benefit judgments suggested by the beneficence model.

The autonomy model insists on respect for the patient's decisions in matters of care. From this point of view, the physician's obligations are not to interfere with the patient's autonomous choices but to assist in their implementation insofar as professional skills and knowledge permit. Like those of the beneficence model, the elements of the autonomy model build on each other to form an interwoven pattern of the moral dimensions of the physician's role—its moral end, its principles, its obligations, and its virtues. These can be represented schematically as follows:

1. *The Moral End of Medicine:* The end of medicine is the promotion of the patient's best interests, as determined by the individual patient's autonomous decisions.
2. *Basic Moral Principle:* The principle of respect for autonomy is the sole fundamental principle. It requires the physician to respect the patient's autonomous decisions and actions regarding medical care.
3. *Derivative Moral Obligations:* From the principle of respect for autonomy the physician's role-related moral obligations are derived: disclosure of medical information, confidentiality, fidelity, and the like.
4. *Derivative Moral Virtues:* From the principle of respect for autonomy the physician's role-related virtues are derived: truthfulness, equanimity, faithfulness, and the like.

Case Applications

We are now in a better position to see how the autonomy model helps Dr. Cox address the moral problem confronting her. Which of the benefits and harms facing Ms. Monroe should be given the greatest weight by Dr. Cox in determining her obligation to Ms. Monroe? The autonomy model insists that goods and harms other than those of the beneficence model must be considered, and it strongly suggests that the greatest weight should be given to Ms. Monroe's decision to accept the risks of laparoscopy and tubal ligation and to forego the possible benefits of continuing on the birth control pill. Just as no appeal to medicine's dissenting view of the patient's best interests can override autonomous choice in this model, so the physician's personal beliefs cannot be overriding. Dr. Cox's personal values of parenthood must play no role in her determination of her obligation to her patient beyond consultation if Ms. Monroe considers and rejects Dr. Cox's values.

Of course, Dr. Cox may protect her autonomy by refusing to comply with Ms. Monroe's request. This can be understood as an appeal to the personal or the professional autonomy of the physician. Any valid appeal to the autonomy rights of the physician will rest on the claim that the physician's basic values and beliefs would be violated by carrying out the patient's request. The patient's autonomy should not be purchased at the price of the physician's personal autonomy. If acceding to a patient's request for medical intervention were to require the physician to act contrary to basic personal values and beliefs, then respect for the physician's autonomy requires that he or she should be free to withdraw from the case and refer the patient to a colleague who does not share those same values and beliefs. This proposal obviously does not imply that such a defense of personal autonomy provides sufficient grounds to tell Ms. Monroe that no physician should perform the sterilization; the argument only offers sufficient reasons to excuse the individual physician from performance of the procedure.

By contrast, any claim to the professional, rather than to the personal autonomy of the physician, may amount to a subtle and unacceptable reassertion of the beneficence model, perhaps even as the *exclusive* moral authority on the best interests of the patient—a moral claim we have undermined throughout the second half of this chapter.

THE TWO MODELS IN CONFLICT

In light of our analysis of the moral problem confronting her, it is evident that Dr. Cox is faced with a genuine moral dilemma. On the one hand, her obligation to her patient under the beneficence model is to refuse to perform the sterilization that Ms. Monroe has requested. On the other hand, Dr. Cox's obligation under the autonomy model is to perform the sterilization as requested. If Dr. Cox acts on the first obligation, she will fail to respect and implement her patient's autonomous decision. If Dr. Cox acts on the second obligation, she will fail to respect and implement medicine's perspective on the risks of medical procedures and their consequences.

The conflict generated by the two models is an inescapable dimension of medical practice: a conflict between the patient's best interests understood from the perspective of medicine and the patient's best interests understood from the perspective of the patient. That conflict is not, as is sometimes thought, an artifact of malpractice suits and contemporary philosophical ethics. Quite the opposite is the case: This conflict is the inevitable result of the histories, traditions, beliefs, and practices in medicine, law, and philosophy that we have traced in this chapter. (However, to say the conflict is inevitable is only to acknowledge its inevitability in *our* social system. That social systems in China, Japan, Bangladesh, and Saudi Arabia may have largely escaped such conflicts is neither a refutation of the claim nor a demonstration that some alternative social system is in some respect preferable to our own and for that reason to be be emulated.)

At this point, the reader may feel frustrated that no definitive and final conclusions have been reached about how Dr. Cox should respond to Ms. Monroe's request for sterilization. It would certainly be satisfying to be able to settle this matter. To do so, however, would be to overlook the normative force of both the beneficence and the autonomy models of moral responsibility. Medicine as known in the West has inherited a complex history, and physicians presently must determine their responsibility to their patients in terms of both models. This is a basic demand in medical ethics because adopting one model *exclusively* will result in the sacrifice of significant values. To use the beneficence model as a trump to override the demands of the autonomy model may result in failure to respect the moral integrity of patients; and to use the autonomy model as a trump to override the demands of the beneficence model may require physicians to act contrary to some of the most basic values of medicine.

The upshot is that the obligations generated by these models are all prima facie, just as all the more general principles mentioned in chapter one generate prima facie obligations. All moral principles seem noble and inviolable when stated free of conflict with other principles. But controversial problems for medical ethics arise when their applicability in circumstances of conflict must be determined. A central task of medical ethics is thus to fix the limits of each of the two models in light of the demands of the other. Because both perspectives merit consideration, discretion is required in clinical decisionmaking. This theme will find a prominent place in subsequent chapters.

Chapter 3

The Management
of Medical Information

In the previous chapter we examined two models of moral responsibility in medicine. In this chapter we apply these models to issues concerning the disclosure of information to patients—an everyday feature of the encounter between physicians and patients and the foundation of effective patient-physician relationships. The issues we shall treat are sometimes expressed in terms of patients' rights, especially rights to an informed consent. However, the term "informed consent" can mislead. It captures only one aspect of informed decisionmaking by patients, namely, decisions that give permission for diagnostic or treatment interventions. In writings on medical ethics, these issues are also sometimes discussed as problems of truth-telling because telling the truth about the patient's condition can conflict with caring for the patient when duties of proper care suggest a suppression of information. However, this labeling is no more satisfactory than the other; it, too, captures only a limited fragment of the problem.

Problems in conveying information to patients also include how to communicate the significance of their presenting complaints, how to maintain effective communication during the process of taking a patient's history and performing a physical examination, and how to explain diagnoses, treatment alternatives, and prognoses.[1] How to preserve autonomous decisionmaking by patients, so that they can make informed decisions, is perhaps the broadest way of stating the problem. To capture the proper scope of information disclosure to patients, we prefer to speak of the "management of medical information," because it emphasizes the physician's role in directing the flow of information to patients.

We shall argue that neither the beneficence model nor the autonomy model is independently sufficient to establish the full range of moral responsibilities involved. In our analysis we often use the law to introduce the problem. This orientation is inescapable because the law has had, and continues to have, a powerful influence on our beliefs about the physician's

---

[1]See Peter B. Heaton, "Negotiation as an Integral Part of the Physician's Clinical Reasoning," *The Journal of Family Practice* 13 (1981): 835–48. See especially his discussion of four stages of negotiation, 846–47.

responsibilities in the management of medical information. However, the law has severe practical limits and is itself shaped by two competing interpretations of human nature that resemble the foundations of the beneficence and autonomy models explored in chapter two. In light of problems physicians and courts alike face in addressing the needs of patients, we argue that both perspectives are essential to an adequate understanding of the physician's responsibilities in managing information.

A CASE STUDY:
HERNIATED DISC INJURY

The following "informed consent" case was ultimately decided in a Los Angeles courtroom in 1970.

In 1961, Bernard Berkey suffered a neck injury, which became aggravated in 1962. Dr. Frank M. Anderson treated him on both occasions and conducted a neurological examination that revealed no obvious problem in the leg or back. Dr. Anderson thought the problem was probably in the neck and suggested a myelogram[2] to see if there was damage to the spinal cord. He said, "We have to get to the bottom of this." Mr. Berkey, according to his sworn and uncontested testimony, asked Dr. Anderson whether the myelogram would be similar to the electromyograms[3] he had undergone. Dr. Anderson responded that myelograms were done for diagnostic and exploratory purposes. He said that patients experience minor discomfort when strapped to a cold table, which then is tilted in various directions to determine the extent of damage to the spinal system. Dr. Anderson was otherwise quite reassuring about the procedure; he said Mr. Berkey would "feel nothing" and promised to order an injection of a pain killer to eliminate any possible discomfort. There was little more to the patient-physician interchange during this discussion. Dr. Anderson did not mention that a myelogram involves a spinal puncture, which is *not* performed in electromyograms.

Dr. Robert E. Rickenberg performed the myelogram procedure, and Mr. Berkey later testified that the following events transpired during the procedure: He first felt a few innocuous "sticks." Then suddenly he felt an

---

[2]"Myelogram" literally means "graph of the spinal cord." During the myelogram, a large gauge, 2½-inch needle is inserted into the lumbar area (lower mid-back) of the spine, while the patient is prone and harnessed on a fluoroscopic table. Eight to ten cc's of spinal fluid are tapped for laboratory analysis, with the needle inserted into the subarachnoid space (just beneath a major covering membrane). An opaque substance (panopaque) is then introduced into the spinal canal through the needle. Tilting the table causes a flow of the substance in the spine, and this flow is captured by X-rays.

[3]An electromyogram is a procedure used to study electrical activity in the muscle, to diagnose a variety of disorders. The procedure involves inserting needle electrodes into muscle tissue. This involves some discomfort, but poses only minor risks.

excruciating pain, as if someone were jamming an ice pick into his lower spine. Mr. Berkey said he had never experienced anything comparable to this pain, which then shot with intensity over his left side and left leg. He "let out a yell," as he later reported, but was told the pain would pass and was sent to rest for 24 hours. When he first stood up he found that he had what he called a "rubber leg": His leg buckled whenever he put weight on it. The next few weeks brought no significant improvement, and he was diagnosed as having "foot drop."[4]

He was examined by several doctors during this period, including Dr. Anderson. One physician, Dr. Faeth, noticed a compression of a nerve, which he judged to be "most probably" caused by a herniated disc.[5] Other possible causes, he later testified, included a tumor, adhesions around the nerve trunk, and the formation of a spur at the margin of the bone. Dr. Anderson was asked in court whether such a herniated disc injury could result from a myelogram. He responded that it could, but only under special circumstances such as "repeated injury with a large bore needle." Dr. Rickenberg testified that he had never heard of anyone developing foot drop as a result of a myelogram.

Mr. Berkey said that nothing whatever had been mentioned to him about the possibility of these levels of pain, injury, and subsequent loss of function. Neither Dr. Anderson nor Dr. Rickenberg had discussed their possible occurrence with Mr. Berkey. Neither physician denied Mr. Berkey's claim to this effect, except to note that they had told him it was a very important diagnostic procedure. Mr. Berkey sued them both—Dr. Rickenberg for negligent performance of the myelogram and Dr. Anderson for a failure to obtain informed consent before ordering the myelogram. The California court that heard an appeal in the case noted that different issues were involved in assessing each physician's actions, but that in each case the court's interest was exclusively in possible damages caused to Mr. Berkey by the responsible physician's action or inaction: "Regarding Dr. Anderson, the questions are whether he obtained the informed consent of his patient before ordering the myelogram and if not, what damages proximately resulted; and as to Dr. Rickenberg, whether there was negligence in administering the myelogram and, if so, whether the injury suffered was the proximate result of such negligence."[6]

The court noted, with regard to the suit against Dr. Anderson, that it is the "duty of a doctor" to explain fully the contemplated procedure and its possible consequences, as well as to obtain the patient's informed consent. If the patient proffered no consent whatever to the myelogram, this omis-

---

[4]"Foot drop" means a falling of the foot because of paralysis of the ankle.

[5]In a herniated disc, the pulpy body at the center of the disc protrudes through the surrounding fibrocartilage, forming a small sac.

[6]*Berkey v. Anderson,* App. 82 Cal. Rptr. 67, p. 72.

sion "would constitute a technical *battery*."[7] If Mr. Berkey had consented, but on the basis of an inadequate disclosure, then Dr. Anderson would be guilty of *negligence*.[8]

To account for some of its reasoning, the court quoted at length a striking passage from a landmark 1957 case—*Salgo v. Leland Stanford, Jr. University Board of Trustees*—which stated that physicians must disclose more to the patients than the mere *nature* of the procedure:

> A physician violates his duty to his patient and subjects himself to liability if he withholds any facts which are necessary to form the basis of an intelligent consent by the patient to the proposed treatment. Likewise the physician may not minimize the known dangers of a procedure or operation in order to induce his patient's consent. At the same time, the physician must place the welfare of his patient above all else and this very fact places him in a position in which he sometimes must choose between two alternative courses of action. One is to explain to the patient every risk attendant upon any surgical procedure or operation, no matter how remote; this may well result in alarming a patient who is already unduly apprehensive and who may as a result refuse to undertake surgery in which there is in fact minimal risk; it may also result in actually increasing the risks by reason of the physiological results of the apprehension itself. The other is to recognize that each patient presents a separate problem, that the patient's mental and emotional condition is important and in certain cases may be crucial, and that in discussing the element of risk a certain amount of discretion must be employed consistent with the full disclosure of facts necessary to an informed consent.[9]

The *Berkey* court then applied parts of this reasoning to the exchange of questions and information between Mr. Berkey and Dr. Anderson:

> Dr. Anderson did not contend that he explained the nature of a myelogram to appellant. . . . The jury could have found that Dr. Anderson gave the appellant no information which would give him any conception of the procedure; in fact, that the information given would have a tendency to mislead the appellant in making his decision. The relationship between a physician and his patient is fiduciary[10] which, like all such relationships, imposes a duty of full disclosure. If appellant was simply told a myelogram was nothing to worry about and that the most uncomfortable thing about it was being tilted about on a cold table, the jury could have concluded that under the facts the statement was actually deceptive. The procedure outlined by the doctors obviously entailed much more, both as to comfort and risk. . . .

---

[7]Battery is an unconsented-to physical violence or constraint inflicted by one person on another.

[8]Negligence is the omission of (or doing of) something that a reasonable person in the circumstances would do (or not do).

[9]*Salgo v. Leland Stanford, Jr. University Board of Trustees*, 154 Cal. App. 2d 560, 578, 317 P.2d 170; as quoted in *Berkey v. Anderson*, p. 77.

[10]A fiduciary relationship is one where a special trust requires scrupulous good faith and candor, including duties to act primarily for another's benefit.

Respondent Anderson further contends that there must be some showing of the requirement in the (physician) community that the patient be advised that some rare and remote result may occur from the procedure followed. He has oversimplified the situation. The question is much broader; not whether he should have informed appellant he might incur a foot drop from the myelogram, but whether the doctor gave him sufficient information as to the nature of a myelogram so that he could intelligently decide whether he wished to have it. If he did not, Dr. Anderson would be liable for all injury appellant sustained in the course of the myelogram, whether the result of negligence or not.[11]

The last part of this passage refers to the nature of the defense offered by Dr. Anderson, who held that other practicing physicians would not have explained such a remote risk of spinal injury under the circumstances and would have routinely ordered the diagnostic procedure. Dr. Anderson and his lawyer argued that this general standard of what other physicians routinely disclose establishes what *should* have been disclosed. Mr. Berkey and his lawyer, by contrast, argued that "the reasonable person's" needs for information set the standard, not simply what the community of physicians actually discloses. The court sided primarily with Mr. Berkey: "A physician's duty to disclose is not governed by the standard practice of the physicians' community, but is a duty imposed by law. . . . To hold otherwise would permit the medical profession to determine its own responsibilities to the patients in a matter of considerable public interest. Further, . . . Dr. Faeth testified that it was not standard practice in obtaining a patient's consent to a myelogram not to inform him that it involves a spinal puncture."[12]

Dr. Anderson's defense of "standard practice" in determining the information that should be released to patients can be understood in terms of the beneficence model. He contends that because the risks of the myelogram are negligible, and because the procedure is such a vital diagnostic tool, doctors who employ this medical technology have determined through clinical experience that they should give the patients minimal information regarding its nature. The implicit assumption is that, from the perspective of medicine, it would actually harm the patient to know more. The dangers are so minimal and its benefits so critical that the added anxiety the patient would experience in knowing these details cannot be justified. Moreover, patients might, out of fear, refuse needed diagnostic or therapeutic interventions. On the other hand, the court views the case in terms of the autonomy model: It was not for the doctor to decide if the benefits of the myelogram were worth the risks involved; that calculation should have been made by the patient, from his own perspective. The doctors had no right to imply that the procedure is simple and painless. Even

[11]*Berkey v. Anderson*, pp. 77–78.
[12]*Berkey v. Anderson*, p. 78.

their goal of helping or curing patients could not justify this apparent disrespect for patient autonomy.

In ruling as it did, the *Berkey* court rejected the view that the level of disclosure of information consistent with a patient's best interests should be determined entirely from the perspective of medicine, even though the *Salgo* court had implied that medical welfare must be placed "above all else." The standard of disclosure for the *Berkey* court is defined by the goal of an "intelligent consent by the patient." That is, appropriate levels of disclosure are to be determined by the information a reasonable patient needs in order to make an informed decision. The *Berkey* court thus seems to discount the important lesson of clinical experience cited by Dr. Anderson—namely, the claim that extensive disclosure can unnecessarily disturb or frighten patients, sometimes leading them to refuse medically indicated diagnostic or therapeutic measures. If this claim is defensible, the "standard of practice of the physicians' community" has a legitimate rationale because it reflects the larger rationale of the beneficence model itself. The court's apparently wholesale rejection of the perspective of the beneficence model may therefore be without merit, as can be seen by examining the history of arguments and certain empirical evidence about the risks and benefits of disclosure.

THE RISKS AND BENEFITS OF DISCLOSURE

In modern medicine the nature and quality of communication in the patient-physician relationship tend to vary with the duration of prior contact, the state of the patient, and how well the physician relates to his or her patient and the patient's family. A patient's right to information ("to know the truth") and the physician's obligation to provide it have traditionally been thought to depend heavily on such situational factors. Most physicians believe that time constraints and other pressing obligations justify departures from such abstract, oversimplified principles as "Don't lie," "Don't deceive," or "Always tell the truth," when used as guides to determine appropriate levels of disclosure. Similarly, few moral philosophers have regarded full, unmonitored disclosure as an absolute physician obligation. The philosopher Henry Sidgwick, for example, argued as follows: "Where deception is designed to benefit the person deceived, Common Sense seems to concede that it may sometimes be right: for example, most persons would not hesitate to speak falsely to an invalid, if this seemed the only way of concealing facts that might produce dangerous shock: nor do I perceive that any one shrinks from telling [certain] fictions to children."[13]

---

[13]Henry Sidgwick, *The Methods of Ethics*, 7th ed. (Indianapolis: Hackett Publishing Co., 1981), p. 316.

A clinically based perspective of this sort powerfully permeates Hippocratic writings in medical ethics, but often the Hippocratic perspective is not properly restrained by the autonomy model. In *On Decorum*, for example, the following admonition appears:

> Perform [the duties of physicians] calmly and adroitly, concealing most things from the patient while you are attending him. Give necessary orders with cheerfulness and sincerity, turning his attention away from what is being done to him; sometimes reprove sharply and emphatically, and sometimes comfort with solicitude and attention, revealing nothing of the patient's future or present condition.[14]

This strategy of nondisclosure or partial disclosure enjoys a prominent place throughout the history of medical ethics.[15] It was adopted in modern times by Thomas Percival[16] and is found in the first Code of Ethics of the American Medical Association.[17]

[14]*On Decorum*. In *Hippocrates*, Vol 2, trans. W. H. S. Jones. (Cambridge, Mass.: Harvard University Press, 1967), pp. 297–99 (from the Loeb editions, 1923–1931). The physician is also advised in Hippocratic writings not to discuss fees during a consultation because it may cause the patient anxieties (*Precepts*, Chapter 6) and because the good physician exhibits a lack of love of money (*On Decorum*, Chapter 5).

[15]See especially Stanley Reiser, "Words as Scalpels: Transmitting Evidence in the Clinical Dialogue," *Annals of Internal Medicine* 92 (1980): 837–42.

[16]Thomas Percival, *Percival's Medical Ethics*, ed. Chauncey Leake (Huntington, N.Y.: Robert E. Krieger Publishing Company, 1975), p. 91:

> A physician should not be forward to make gloomy prognostications, because they savor of empiricism, by magnifying the importance of his services in the treatment or cure of the disease. But he should not fail, on proper occasions, to give to the friends of the patient, timely notice of danger, when it really occurs, and even to the patient himself, if absolutely necessary. This office, however, is so peculiarly alarming, when executed by him, that it ought to be declined, whenever it can be assigned to any other person of sufficient judgment and delicacy. For the physician should be the minister of hope and comfort to the sick; that by such cordials to the drooping spirit, he may smooth the bed of death, revive expiring life, and counteract the depressing influence of those maladies which rob the philosopher of fortitude, and the Christian of consolation.

[17]American Medical Association, "Code of Medical Ethics," in *Proceedings of the National Convention, 1846–1847* (Chicago: American Medical Association, 1847), reprinted in Stanley Reiser et al., *Ethics in Medicine* (Cambridge, Mass.: MIT Press, 1977), p. 29.

> A physician should not be forward to make gloomy prognostications, because they savour of empiricism, by magnifying the importance of his services in the treatment or cure of the disease. But he should not fail, on proper occasions, to give to the friends of the patient timely notice of danger, when it really occurs; and even to the patient himself, if absolutely necessary. This office, however, is so peculiarly alarming when executed by him, that it ought to be declined whenever it can be assigned to any other person of sufficient judgment and delicacy. For, the physician should be the minister of hope and comfort to the sick; that, by such cordials to the drooping spirit, he may smooth the bed of death, revive expiring life, and counteract the depressing influence of those maladies which often disturb the tranquility of the most resigned, in their last moments. The life of a sick person can be shortened not only by the acts, but also by the words or the manner of a physician. It is, therefore, a sacred duty to guard himself carefully in this respect, and to avoid all things which have a tendency to discourage the patient and to depress his spirits.

The principal worry expressed in these historical writings about disclosures is that information might be harmful rather than helpful to seriously ill patients. For example, patients may become agitated as a consequence of full disclosure, sometimes leading to more complicated courses of recovery. This venerable hypothesis has its contemporary adherents, as the following influential statement by Elizabeth F. Loftus and James F. Fries indicates:

> A considerable body of psychological evidence indicates that humans are highly suggestible. Information has been found to change people's attitudes, to change their moods and feelings, and even to make them believe they have experienced events that never in fact occurred. This alone would lead one to suspect that adverse reactions might result from information given during an informed consent discussion.
>
> An examination of the medical evidence demonstrates that . . . not only can positive therapeutic effects be achieved by suggestion, but negative side effects and complications can similarly result. For example, among subjects who participated in a drug study after the usual informed consent procedure, many of those given an injection of a placebo reported physiologically unlikely symptoms such as dizziness, nausea, vomiting, and even mental depressions. One subject given the placebo reported that these effects were so strong that they caused an automobile accident. Many other studies provide similar data indicating that to a variable but often scarifying degree, explicit suggestion of possible adverse effects causes subjects to experience these effects. Recent hypotheses that heart attack may follow coronary spasm indicate physiological mechanisms by which explicit suggestions, and the stress that may be produced by them, might prove fatal. Thus, the possible consequences of suggested symptoms range from minor annoyance to, in extreme cases, death.
>
> If protection of the subject is the reason for obtaining informed consent, the possibility of iatrogenic harm [harm caused by a physician's treatment] to the subject as a direct result of the consent ritual must be considered.[18]

A recent Presidential Commission investigated such claims and concluded as follows: "Despite all the anecdotes about patients who committed suicide, suffered heart attacks, or plunged into prolonged depression upon being told 'bad news,' little documentation exists for claims that informing patients is more dangerous to their health than not informing them, particularly when the informing is done in a sensitive and tactful fashion.

---

[18]Elizabeth F. Loftus and James F. Fries, "Informed Consent May be Hazardous to Health," *Science* 204 (6 April 1979): 11. The position and argument of Loftus and Fries have been subjected to important criticism. See Ruth Barcan Marcus, Bruce Kuklick, and Sacvan Bercovitch, Letter, *Science* 205 (17 August 1979): 644. These authors have shown its logical flaws, while important empirical limitations have been pointed to by Ruth Faden et al., "Disclosures of Information to Patients in Medical Care," *Medical Care* 19 (July 1981): 718–33, esp. 731, and Ruth Faden et al., "Disclosure Standards and Informed Consent," *Journal of Health Politics, Policy, and Law* 6 (1981): 255–84. Faden et al. show that there exists better evidence for the Loftus-Fries position than they themselves adduce, but that there exists equally powerful counterevidence.

... There is much to suggest that therapeutic privilege has been vastly overused."[19]

Despite this cloud over the claims, physicians continue to report that many of their sick and dependent patients often find extensive disclosures of potential hazards frightening and incomprehensible. For example, Dr. Robert M. Soule, in response to Sissela Bok's views on lying to patients, argues as follows:

> She states there is no evidence that total candor does any harm to patients. Clinical experience simply doesn't bear this out. . . . Through the years I have seen too many examples of the lethal effect of total candor, including mental breakdowns and suicides by patients given a cold-turkey diagnosis.
> Years ago a Harvard report documented fatal ventricular fibrillation brought on by fright in healthy people. And a letter in the May 12, 1977, *New England Journal of Medicine*, cited two heart attackes—one fatal—after patients with no history of cardiac disease had been given full information for consent to noncardiac surgery. The authors said patients often complained they "could not sleep all night before their procedure because of preoccupation and concern." . . .
> Many times a conference with the family suggests a patient needs to be protected from the "whole truth." . . .
> In a crisis many people would prefer compassion to total frankness, which can have a devastating emotional impact.[20]

Although it is still uncertain under what conditions and to what extent full disclosure for the sake of informed consent can become harmful to a patient's health,[21] it is documented beyond reasonable doubt that physicians do routinely withhold information when they believe excessive fright or serious risk to the patient would result from a disclosure. For example, a carefully structured study examined practices of disclosure by neurologists. Almost twenty percent of sampled neurologists reported that they routinely suppress information about the consequences of taking the drug Dilantin[22] when they believe their patients would become upset by the information.[23] It is not clear, however, that the public in general disagrees

[19]President's Commission for the Study of Ethical Problems in Medicine and Biomedicine and Behavioral Research, *Making Health Care Decisions: The Ethical and Legal Implications of Informed Consent in the Patient-Practitioner Relationship* (Washington: U.S. Government Printing Office, 1982), vol. 1, p. 96.

[20]Robert M. Soule, "The Case Against 'Total Candor'," *Medical World News* 20 (14 May 1979): 94.

[21]The inconclusiveness of presently available evidence is surveyed in Alan Meisel and Loren Roth, "What We Do and Do Not Know About Informed Consent," *Journal of the American Medical Association* 246 (27 November 1981): 2473–77. See also the summary evidence of a survey performed by Louis Harris and Associates, in President's Commission, *Making Health Care Decisions*, pp. 96–102.

[22]Dilantin is a drug used to control seizures. The drug's side effects include slurred speech, dizziness, nausea, vomiting, measles-like rash, and, for pregnant women, the risk of birth defects in offspring.

[23]Faden et al., "Disclosures of Information to Patients in Medical Care," esp. 726, 731.

with these practices of physician discretion in the monitoring of information. In the aforementioned study by a Presidential Commission, fifty-six percent of the public expressed a belief that some patients should be told less about their treatment than other patients.[24]

It is a matter of overwhelming importance that any generalizations from such data about physician behavior and patients' attitudes reflect the type of illness and degree of morbidity, as well as the context in which disclosures are made and the background of the patients involved. If a healthy patient wants information about the side effects of a prescribed drug or a parent seeks the results of a pediatrician's examination of a young child, we would not expect and would quickly condemn nondisclosure of relevant information. In such instances, a physician can relate to a patient or parent without the degree of emotional dependence that inevitably accompanies the state of sickness. Information can be freely dispatched without fear of undue alarm, let alone terror.

However, many patients with diseases such as metastatic cancer or end-stage kidney disease face life-threatening circumstances that may inherently involve choices among alternative courses of treatment, each carrying terrifying risks. Here, any physician must employ managerial skills, taking into account the patient's need for information and ability to deal with it—as, for example, when the terminally ill cancer patient cannot accept the fact that his or her death is imminent, and thus refuses palliative treatment. Is it a primary responsibility of the physician to inform the patient that he or she has but a few months to live? Or is this only a rather wooden way of discharging legal responsibilities while failing the patient at a deeper moral level—for example, failing to help the patient come to grips with his or her mortality and the impact of his or her death on family and friends?

Both empirical evidence and philosophical argument suggest that considerations of risks and benefits of disclosure, as understood through the beneficence model, play an appropriate role in the physician's determination of moral responsibility. The perspective of medicine is invoked to determine the relative weight of harm full disclosure causes to some patients: They might refuse needed diagnostic or therapeutic interventions, suffer unnecessarily, or have more complicated courses of recovery. The physician assumes an obligation to avoid these harms while providing the benefits of medical care. Dr. Anderson's behavior in the diagnosis of Mr. Berkey's condition reflects this approach, even if his execution of it is flawed.

In previous chapters we witnessed a similar approach to the physician's obligations by examining traditional sources of medical ethics. An obligation of strict disclosure was advocated by Dr. Bard (see pp. 15–16), while discretion on the part of the physician to protect the patient from harm was

---

[24]President's Commission, *Making Health Care Decisions*, p. 72.

defended by Dr. Hooker (see pp. 15–16). We also saw that a separate line of argument has been used in the history of medical ethics that appeals more vigorously to the autonomy model. Dr. Cabot's views, for example, go further by providing an "experiment of telling the truth." In Cabot's experience, significant harm is not done to patients or their families by truthful disclosure in diagnosis, prognosis, and treatment: "I will sum up the results of my experiments with truth and falsehood, by saying that I have not yet found any case in which a lie does not do more harm than good, and by expressing my belief that if everyone will carefully repeat the experiments he will reach similar results. The technic of truth-telling is sometimes difficult, perhaps more difficult than the technic of lying, but its results make it worth acquiring."[25]

Cabot's beliefs are reflected, belatedly, in surveys showing a recent and dramatic shift in physician's behavior in disclosing diagnoses to cancer patients. Whereas twenty years ago most physicians (88%) did not disclose the diagnosis of cancer,[26] most physicians (98%) now report making routine and generally complete disclosures.[27] Evidence has also been adduced to show that not only is disclosure not necessarily harmful, it can prove to be of positive benefit to patients and their families. In a study of pediatric cancer patients, a team from the Sidney Farber Cancer Institute and Children's Hospital in Boston reports that early disclosure of cancer diagnoses tends to benefit patients and reduces stress and anxiety during treatment and long-term recovery.[28] Here, the patient's subjective responses are invoked to show that disclosure is not harmful, is often beneficial, and is preferred by patients and their families. In the previously cited study of disclosure about the risks of Dilantin, one hundred percent of the patients who had taken the drug, and who therefore were familiar with its consequences, wanted to be told the information about its risks by their physician, even if that information might make them upset or anxious.[29]

Another study shows that patients rate their satisfaction with the patient-physician relationship more highly if their physician manages information with an accent on disclosure. This is especially true for anxious patients: "The physician who gives verbal attention to the patient's problem by taking time to understand and answer questions, give explanations, and show

[25]Richard Clarke Cabot, "The Use of Truth and Falsehood in Medicine," *American Medicine* 5 (1903): 344–49, in Stanley Reiser et al., *Ethics in Medicine*, pp. 219–20.

[26]Donald Oken, "What to Tell Cancer Patients: A Study of Medical Attitudes," *Journal of the American Medical Association* 175 (1961): 1120–28. See also W. D. Kelly and S. R. Friesen, "Do Cancer Patients Want to be Told?" *Surgery* 27 (1950): 822–26.

[27]D. H. Novack, E. J. Freireich, and S. Vaisrub, "Changes in Physicians' Attitudes Toward Telling the Cancer Patient," *Journal of the American Medical Association* 241 (1979): 897–900. Questions have been raised about the methodological adequacy of all these surveys.

[28]L. A. Slavin et al., "Communication of the Cancer Diagnosis to Pediatric Patients: Impact on Long-Term Adjustment," *American Journal of Psychiatry* 139 (February 1982): 182.

[29]Faden et al., "Disclosures of Information to Patients in Medical Care," esp. 726, 731.

a friendly interest in the patient has a satisfying effect, and may have a psychologically therapeutic effect, on that patient."[30] If the patient's perspective is the basis for determining the weight of the harms and goods of disclosure, as the autonomy model insists, then the physician would seem obligated to disclose information to patients.

Review of argument and evidence on both sides thus indicates that the basic issue in the management of medical information is how the physician should balance the goods and harms of various levels of disclosure. Under the professional community standard, as invoked by Dr. Anderson, the rationale is that of the beneficence model: Medicine's perspective should be used to determine the weight of the harms and goods of disclosure. By contrast, the *Berkey* court insisted that the perspective of the informed patient should determine the appropriate weighting—an approach that reflects the autonomy model. Because both perspectives have merit, we should expect that neither the law nor medical ethics will settle finally on a single directive. As we shall now see, the legal history of which *Berkey* is a key part does *not* result in the complete triumph of the patient-based perspective over the professionally based one. The result, instead, is a delicate tension in the law between the two perspectives.

LEGAL REQUIREMENTS

Legal History of the Informed Consent Doctrine

The law of informed consent is still actively evolving. As the *Berkey* court noted, its early foundations are in tort law of battery, which holds that an individual can be validly "touched" by another only when he or she authorizes that touching. When touching is nonauthorized, questions of liability for the causal outcome are raised. This legal doctrine of informed consent has passed through three identifiable stages in the United States, each demarcated by landmark legal decisions.

The 1914–1957 Period. The first phase ran roughly from 1914 to 1957—a period characterized by concern about whether a patient had given a consent that acknowledged some general description of the procedure involved. The most influential case was *Schloendorff v. Society of New York Hospitals* (1914).[31] A fibroid tumor had been removed from the abdomen of a female patient, but the patient had requested "no operation." The

---

[30]S. A. Wartman et al., "Do Prescriptions Adversely Affect Doctor-Patient Interactions?" *American Journal of Public Health* 71 (1981): 1360.

[31]*Schloendorff v. Society of New York Hospitals*, 105 N.E. 92 (1914). Ironically, this landmark case pertained to hospital liability, and the court found neither a violation of informed consent nor even delivered its findings in terms of consent.

court cited negligence and trespass in noting that the tumor had been removed "without her consent or knowledge." Justice Cardozo—as quoted in chapter two—vigorously insisted on the patient's right to self-determination and on the liability of the physician when patients are not given the opportunity to exercise that right by consenting to treatment. Subsequent cases between 1914 and 1957 exhibit a consistent pattern of reasoning in the courts: Either a patient consented or failed to consent; a partial or incomplete consent plays no role in the court's decision. This analysis sprang from the prevalent notion at the time that consents were broad; a simple, routine disclosure was given about the procedure itself, usually without much background explanation.

The 1957–1972 Period.   The second phase involved a transition from the bare fact of consent to a concern about the quality of consent, with a special emphasis on the quality of disclosure. The *Berkey v. Anderson* case mentioned earlier was in litigation during the early days of this period, and was decided near its conclusion. In this legal environment, the term "informed consent" was born and flourished, and the legal category of "professional negligence" came to describe a wrong caused by a failure to inform *adequately*. The following aspects of the legal doctrine stabilized: As the *Berkey* court noted, battery is involved if a procedure is performed without basic disclosure as to nature and scope prior to consent (whether by omission or misrepresentation). One is battered when even simple consent is not present, or when a "consent" is vitiated by misrepresentation. Simple consent is regarded as a necessary first level of any valid consent. Negligence, by contrast, is involved when a procedure is performed with consent based on disclosure as to its nature and scope (and so there *is* simple consent), but without disclosure as to possible complications or risks of the procedure and possible alternatives to it. (Battery involves injuries as the result of intended action, whereas no intent is required in negligence.)

Thus, during the 1957 to 1972 period a more complex consent requirement emerged. It established a second level of valid consent. This conclusion is embraced by the *Berkey* court and was one important reason Dr. Anderson was found guilty of negligence. Beginning in the late 1950s, the courts began to consider informed consent a matter of professional conduct and to establish the breach of a duty to inform as negligence—not battery—therefore aligning informed consent cases with other medical malpractice cases.[32]

[32]First in 1957 with *Salgo v. Leland Stanford, Jr. University Board of Trustees,* 154 Cal. App. 2d 560, 317 P.2d 170 (1957). For legal details including explanations of the shifts discussed here, see *Trogun v. Fruchtman,* 58 Wis. 2d 596, pp. 599–600, 207 N.W. 2d 297, p. 313 (1973); Alan McCoid, "A Reappraisal of Liability for Unauthorized Medical Treatment," *Minnesota Law Review* 41 (1957): 381, 423–25; James Ludlam, *Informed Consent* (Chicago: American Hospital Association, 1978); and Alan Meisel, "Expansion of Liability for Medical Accidents: From Negligence to Strict Liability by Way of Informed Consent," *Nebraska Law Review* 56

The courts applied this approach even in cases where there was no dispute about whether the level of disclosure was consistent with sound medical practice—a matter at issue in *Berkey*. An important case was *Natanson v. Kline,* a 1960 Kansas case in which cobalt radiation therapy was administered after a radical mastectomy to the area where the cancer had been removed. Injuries to the chest, skin, and cartilage resulted from the radiation therapy, and the woman brought suit against her physician. The physician acknowledged that risks were inherent in the procedure, but he "failed to warn the patient of risks of (such) bodily injury." A trial court found for the pysicians, but an appeals court asserted that physicians are required to disclose the nature, dangers, and probable consequences of cobalt radiation and may not substitute even *sound* medical judgment for the patient's judgment. Consequently, the appeals court judge viewed the protection of autonomy as the major purpose of informed consent and denied that the patient's medical best interests could legitimately override duties of disclosure.

Natanson not only established a category of "risks" that must be disclosed to the patient, but also established that mere consent does not shield the physician from negligence (liability for injury), even if the medical performance is good. That is, the medical practice can be flawless, but if injury results from a routine risk, and the risk was not disclosed, the physician is liable. The "consent" was invalidated in *Natanson* because the patient was not informed of those "collateral hazards" any "reasonable medical practitioner" would disclose.[33]

The Post-1972 Period. When the *Berkey* court rejected Dr. Anderson's argument that the standards determining his disclosure obligation to the patient were set by what physicians routinely disclose about risks, it was knocking on the door of some newly emerging problems. Since 1972, several influential courts have addressed the issue of what counts as adequate disclosure, in light of the patient-centered standard established in some courts during the 1957 to 1972 period. The 1972 cases that have achieved landmark status are *Canterbury v. Spence* and *Cobbs v. Grant.*[34] Let us first briefly examine these important cases and certain problems about disclosure standards that they create. We shall then offer some reservations— mainly moral reservations—about their disclosure requirements.

(1977). The informed consent action in negligence has five elements: (1) the physician's *duty* to give information (under the appropriate informational standard) which is part of his professional duty of due care; (2) *breach of duty;* (3) *risk:* materialization of the undisclosed outcome or possible outcome; (4) *proximate causation:* had a plaintiff been informed of an outcome or risk he or she would not have consented; (5) damages, i.e., *actual injury.* If the plaintiff can prove the existence of all five elements, the physician is liable for medical malpractice, regardless of the skill with which treatment was provided.

[33]*Natanson v. Kline,* 350 P.2d 1093 (1960).

[34]*Canterbury v. Spence,* 464 F.2d 772 (1972); *Cobbs v. Grant,* 502 P.2d 1 (1972).

Canterbury v. Spence was the first and most influential of the landmark informed consent cases in this period. This case involved a laminectomy[35] for severe back pain. Subsequent to the laminectomy, the patient fell from a hospital bed, a fall that caused major paralysis. The patient had not been warned that a laminectomy might increase the danger of paralysis as the result of such events as falling out of bed. A second operation failed to relieve the paralysis, and an appeals court held that risk of possible paralysis should have been disclosed prior to the first procedure. Judge Spottswood Robinson's opinion focused on autonomy: "The root premise is the concept, fundamental in American jurisprudence, that 'every human being of adult years and sound mind has a right to determine what shall be done with his own body.' . . . "[36] True consent was held in this case to be contingent upon the informed exercise of a choice; thus, the physician's disclosure should have provided the patient an opportunity to assess available options and attendant risks, such as paralysis. As to sufficiency of information, the court held: "The patient's right of self-decision shapes the boundaries of the duty to reveal. That right can be effectively exercised only if the patient possesses enough information to enable an intelligent choice."[37]

Cobbs v. Grant came to similar conclusions. The court required disclosure of "*all* significant perils pertaining to death or serious harm," and rejected the view that decisions whether to proceed with a specific therapy are solely medical determinations. The court insisted that all significant risks peculiar to a proposed procedure must be divulged, as judged by the extent to which a prudent or reasonable person in the patient's position would want to know about the risk. In this case, Dr. F. P. Grant examined Mr. Ralph Cobbs and diagnosed a duodenal ulcer. Surgery was recommended, and Dr. Grant explained the *nature* of the operation to Mr. Cobbs, but did not discuss any of several complicated *risks* inherent in the surgery itself. Mr. Cobbs consented to the operation and an apparently successful surgery was performed. But complications arose: Mr. Cobbs suffered intense abdominal pain, injuries to the spleen that necessitated a subsequent operation, and a developing gastric ulcer. All are risks inherent in surgery performed to relieve a duodenal ulcer. The court declared these events "links in a chain of low probability events inherent in the initial operation," and reasoned that Dr. Grant's failure to disclose them ran contrary to the physician's duty to disclose.

These two cases inaugurated the present period, and many courts now require disclosures as to a medical diagnosis, prognosis with and without treatment, proposed treatments, risks inherent in the treatment, and

---

[35]A laminectomy is the surgical removal of parts of the vertebrae, commonly including spinous processes of the vertebrae.

[36]From *Canterbury*, p. 786, quoting *Schloendorff v. Society of New York Hospitals.*

[37]*Canterbury v. Spence*, p. 786 (footnotes omitted).

alternative treatment modes and their risks. Such disclosure requirements have met with opposition in much of the medical community. The following reaction by Dr. Robert B. Howard is typical:

> Is it good medical practice to discuss with an apprehensive, febrile, partially obtunded patient with pneumonia the possibility that the medication selected may produce an anaphylactoid reaction or may cause exfoliative dermatitis, urticaria, serum sickness, fever, hemolytic anemia, leukopenia, thrombocytopenia, neuropathy, and/or nephropathy? Must I explain all of these and present optional forms of therapy, each of which has its own list of possible side effects?
> I believe that such action on my part would be inappropriate and irresponsible. Yet, if I interpret correctly the recent court decisions and awards, my failure to discuss even the rarest potential adverse reactions may expose me to successful legal action if such reaction occurs.
> I believe that truly informed consent is an impossible goal in many, indeed most, of our daily clinical experiences. I believe that with each patient we must use our best professional judgment to guide the discussion—the disease, the patient's immediate clinical condition and intellectual capacity, and the actual probability of adverse events connected with treatment all are pertinent. Obtaining informed consent that meets strict legal requirements will solve few health care problems and will seriously impede recovery in many cases.[38]

The requirements denounced in this critique have gradually crept up on medicine, which has witnessed a shift from a beneficence-based standard of disclosure to the autonomy-based standard present in the 1972 cases. A professionally based standard of disclosure has its source in the beneficence model, while a patient-based standard of disclosure fits with the values in the autonomy model. This may be seen more clearly if we structure what we have learned about legal history in terms specific to the *standards* governing physician disclosure that we discussed previously. We make this effort not with the intent to reform the law, but rather to construct an adequate general standard for clinical practice from the moral point of view.

Standards Governing Physician Disclosure

The Professional Practice Standard. A professional practice standard was invoked by Dr. Anderson in the *Berkey* case and traditionally has been the standard of disclosure favored by physicians and others favoring the beneficence model. The professional practice standard holds that adequate disclosure is determined by the customary rules or traditional practices of the professional community of physicians, who are presumed to be in a privileged position to determine their patients' best interests. The physician, by reference to the perspective of medicine—specifically, by reference to the

---

[38]Robert B. Howard, "More on Informed Consent," *Postgraduate Medicine* 65 (January 1979): 25.

practice of physicians in general—determines the balance of harms and goods of disclosure and establishes both the topics to be discussed and the amount and kinds of information to be disclosed about each topic. The disclosure needing to be made (if any) is as much a professional decision as the physician's original diagnosis.[39] Thus, the burden of proof in most legal jurisdictions is on the patient to show that the physician's disclosure failed to conform to established standards.

Many problems, however, attend this professional practice standard for disclosure. First, as the *Canterbury* and *Cobbs* courts noted, it is unclear that customary standards for disclosure prevail in the medical profession, and in any event, the rules that would constitute the standard are not precisely formulated.[40] Hence, it is difficult to answer questions about how much consensus is necessary—and within which fields of medicine—in order to establish that a medical practice standard for disclosure does in fact exist. Moreover, if custom alone is decisive, then negligent disclosures are "acceptable" if physicians generally provide inferior information and precautions.[41] Finally, the professional practice standard neglects the patient's autonomy rights in the face of no empirical evidence that physicians make either good decisions about appropriate information or even that they have a better conception of what is in a patient's best interest than does the patient. Critics of this first standard hold that weighing the harms and goods of disclosure is not a medical skill to be measured by a professional standard; rather it is an individual value judgment reserved to the affected person alone. This perspective is clearly operative in Mr. Berkey's argument.

The Reasonable Person Standard.   In the aftermath of *Canterbury,* the reasonable person standard has emerged as a prominent legal criterion. This standard was implicitly invoked by Mr. Berkey, even though his case antedated *Canterbury.* Approximately twenty-five percent of the legal jurisdictions in the United States now accept this new criterion, while the remaining seventy-five percent still adhere to the more traditional medical practice standard. Thus, while there has been a significant shift toward a patient-based standard, that shift has yet to be accepted in the majority of legal jurisdictions.

According to the reasonable person standard, which flows from the legal principle of respect for self-determination, the physician must disclose to

---

[39]See Marcus Plant, "The Decline of Informed Consent," *Washington and Lee Law Review* 35 (1978): 96–99.

[40]Alan Stone notes—in "Informed Consent: Special Problems for Psychiatry," *Hospital and Community Psychiatry* 30 (May 1979): 322, and "Reply," *Hospital and Community Psychiatry* 30 (September 1979): 637—that physicians are not trained uniformly in appropriate disclosures. He expresses doubt that "any such standard exists" (p. 323).

[41]See Jon R. Waltz, "The Rise and Gradual Fall of the Locality Rule in Medical Malpractice Litigation," *DePaul Law Review* 18 (1969), esp. p. 408.

the patient all information relevant to a decision, as judged by what a hypothetical reasonable person would want to know. Providing material information is part of the physician's fiduciary duty of due care, and a physician's medical expertise is recognized as only one of several factors that a patient may wish to take into consideration. The relevance of a piece of information to a patient's decision is measured not by a professional judgment, but instead by the significance a reasonable person would attach to a risk in reaching a decision. If that risk would be regarded as significant, it should be disclosed. If not, disclosure is unnecessary. Therefore, in theory, a physician may be found guilty of negligent disclosure even if the physician's behavior conforms perfectly to recognized and routine professional practice (as occurred in *Natanson*).

Whatever its virtues, the reasonable person standard harbors problems. First, the concept of the "materiality" or relevance of information is only ambiguously defined in *Canterbury* and related cases, and the central concept of "the reasonable person" goes altogether undefined. Second, no specific or extensive duty of disclosure follows from such a standard; thus, from the perspective of autonomy, the "new" standard expressed in *Canterbury* may give a false sense of an advance over the older standard. Indeed, some empirical evidence suggests that in medical practice it makes no difference in physicians' behavior in making disclosures whether the medical practice standard or the reasonable person standard is operative in the relevant legal jurisdiction.[42] Finally, because application of the abstract reasonable person standard to a concrete case would require reference to specific facts of the case, an unresolved problem is how to understand what information the reasonable person would want "under the same or similar circumstances" as those of the patient. If, for example, a physician fails to disclose a remote risk of surgery, we must ask whether a reasonable person in this patient's *precise* position would have wanted to be told of the risk. But how broadly is *that* position to be described? This leads to consideration of a third standard, which has been proposed to answer this question.

The Subjective Standard. Individual patients have different needs for information, especially if they have idiosyncratic or unique beliefs, deviant health behaviors, a unique family or personal history, or the like. Such patients require a different informational base than that required by most persons. For example, Mr. Berkey's possible confusion of a myelogram with the electromyogram with which he had first-hand familiarity suggests a need to explain the myelogram in different terms than those used to explain the procedure to another patient who had never undergone an electromyogram (at least by pointing out that there is no similarity between the two). Such special circumstances are clearly relevant to the process of

---

[42]See the two studies by Faden et al., "Disclosures of Information to Patients in Medical Care" and "Disclosure Standards and Informed Consent."

decisionmaking. If a physician has grounds for believing that a patient needs such information, the autonomy model strongly suggests its disclosure. By thus following the demands of this model, the reasonable person standard is modified to a "subjective" form.[43]

The subjective standard has been rejected almost wholly by the courts,[44] largely because of the legal doctrine of proximate cause on which so many informed consent malpractice cases turn. According to the proximate cause theory, a patient cannot recover for injury unless he or she can show that the physician's negligence in disclosing information was a proximate cause of the injury. There is no causal connection in law between a physician's negligent disclosure and the patient's injury unless consent would *not* have been given had a proper disclosure been made. If a subjective approach were taken to the proximate cause issue, a patient could recover if *that particular* patient would not have consented had an adequate disclosure been made. *Canterbury* and other courts insist that this determination would be guesswork and constantly would place physicians in jeopardy of the vindictive hindsight of patients, including possible outright falsification. Hence, these courts allow only the "objective reasonable person" to be the appropriate standard.

Such *legal* arguments fail to determine whether the subjective standard is a better *moral* standard for communications in the patient-physician relationship. As we shall now see, this standard is strongly recommended from the point of view of morality.

COMPETING MODELS
OF DECISIONAL AUTHORITY

Jay Katz, professor of law and psychiatry at Yale, has written extensively on problems of legal standards of disclosure and their inadequacies. He has convincingly argued that the primary problem underlying the aforementioned battles over shifting legal standards is not one that the law directly addresses or is well equipped to address. The fundamental question, he

---

[43]For legal commentary favoring this standard, see Alexander Capron, "Informed Consent in Catastrophic Disease Research and Treatment," *University of Pennsylvania Law Review* 123 (1974): 364–76; L. W. Kessenick and P. A. Mankin, "Medical Malpractice: The Right to be Informed," *University of San Francisco Law Review* 8 (1973); Marcus Plant, "An Analysis of Informed Consent," *Fordham Law Review* 36 (1968); and Leonard L. Riskin, "Informed Consent: Looking for the Action," *University of Illinois Law Forum 1975* (1975). The standard has been overtly embraced as a moral standard for medical practice by Charles Culver and Bernard Gert, *Philosophy in Medicine: Conceptual and Ethical Issues in Medicine and Psychiatry* (New York: Oxford University Press, 1982), Chapter 3.

[44]At least one court—the Oklahoma Supreme Court—has adopted a subjective approach. See *Scott v. Bradford*, 606 P.2d 554 (Okla. 1980), esp. 556 and the analysis of this case in "Note," *Tulsa Law Journal* 15 (1980): 665ff.

holds, is "Whose judgment is to be respected and overriding?" Katz has approached the prevailing situations in law and medicine through what he calls a "conflict between two visions": a "vision of human beings as autonomous persons and . . . deference to paternalism, another powerful vision of man's interaction with man."[45] "Autonomous persons" here refers to an individual's capacity to assume authority over his or her medical fate. This capacity law and medicine alike sometimes recognize as the patient's right to self-determination and consequent right to the fullest possible disclosure—an autonomy-based standard. "Paternalism" here means that the physician assumes authority to manage the information disclosed, without consulting the patient, on grounds of beneficence.

Katz notes that the courts have traditionally paid allegiance to this vision of humans as autonomous only to deviate from their pronouncements once the realities of medical practice and the patient's decisionmaking capacities in medical facilities are brought to the court's attention. Katz therefore sees the entire legal doctrine of informed consent—including all the standards discussed above—as little more than a symbol of the need for patient decisionmaking—a symbol having virtually no impact on how decisions are made by patients, courts, or physicians:

> The conflict created by uncertainties about the extent to which individual and societal well-being is better served by encouraging patients' self-determination or supporting physicians' paternalism is the central problem of informed consent. This fundamental conflict, reflecting a thoroughgoing ambivalence about human beings' capacities for taking care of themselves and need for care-taking, has shaped judicial pronouncements on informed consent more decisively than is commonly appreciated. The assertion of a 'need' for physicians' discretion—for a professional expert's rather than a patient's judgment as to what constitutes well-being—reveals this ambivalence. Other oft-invoked impediments to fostering patients' self-determination, such as patients' medical ignorance, doctors' precious time, the threat of increased litigation, or the difficulty of proving what actually occurred in the dialogue between physician and patient are, substantially, rationalizations which obscure the basic conflict over whose judgment is to be respected.[46]

The lengthy quotation in *Berkey* of the 1957 precedent case *Salgo v. Leland Stanford, Jr. University Board of Trustees* (see p. 55) can be used to illustrate Katz's valuable contentions. The *Salgo* court notes that *any* withholding of facts "necessary to form the basis of an intelligent consent by the patient" is a violation of a physician's duty to the patient. Having made this strong pronouncement, the court does an immediate about-face that deserves quotation for a second time: The "patient's mental and emotional

---

[45]Jay Katz, "Informed Consent—A Fairy Tale? Law's Vision," *University of Pittsburgh Law Review* 39 (Winter 1977): 139.

[46]Ibid.

condition is important and in certain cases may be crucial, and . . . in discussing the element of risk a certain amount of discretion must be employed consistent with the full disclosure of facts necessary to an informed consent."[47]

The need in many cases of physician discretion, under the ideal of a fiduciary relationship between patient and physician, leads the court to hold that on the one hand, an autonomy-based standard of disclosure sometimes justifiably yields to a beneficence-based standard, and on the other hand, a beneficence-based standard sometimes justifiably yields to an autonomy-based one. Moreover, the court suggests that a physician *violates a duty* and invites a malpractice suit by not providing sufficient information on which to base an intelligence choice; at the same time, the court suggests that the duty itself is *validly qualified* by the physician's professional discretion. Hence, Katz properly doubts that there can be complete consistency between "physician discretion" in the disclosure of information and "full disclosure of facts." "Only in dreams or fairy tales," he writes, "can 'discretion' to withhold crucial information so easily and magically be reconciled with 'full disclosure'."[48] *Salgo* and virtually all subsequent courts have exhibited such wishful thinking.

The law thus seems committed to two competing moral objectives. The first is that patients should be treated as autonomous, with the right to make informed decisions. The second is that it is appropriate for the physician to limit disclosure depending on the weight of the harms and goods of disclosure. When the law focuses on patient autonomy, the emphasis is on decisionmaking by patients; when the law focuses on the possible consequences of full disclosure to patients, as understood from medicine's perspective, the emphasis is on professional discretion and the avoidance of harm to patients. Physicians are to respect autonomy, but they also may validly invoke a "therapeutic privilege"—one that permits physicians on grounds of "good medical practice" not to disclose information (to the patient, anyway) if it would "seriously jeopardize the recovery of an unstable, temperamental, or severely depressed patient."[49] Because courts must eventually evaluate a broad range of problems in managing information, they have not been able to escape confrontation with the full power of the

---

[47]*Salgo*, as quoted in *Berkey v. Anderson*, p. 72.

[48]Katz, "Informed Consent—A Fairy Tale?": 138 (see also 150), and "Disclosure and Consent in Psychiatric Practice: Mission Impossible?" in *Law and Ethics in the Practice of Psychiatry*, ed. Charles Hofling (New York: Brunner-Mazel, Inc., 1981), p. 93.

[49]*Natanson v. Kline*, p. 1103. For slightly different formulations, see *Sard v. Hardy*, 367 A.2d, p. 1022 and *Canberbury v. Spence*, p. 789. Even here, however, considerable uncertainty surrounds the precise conditions under which therapeutic privilege may be validly invoked, the courts having left indeterminate *how* adverse the impact of disclosed information must be and how much latitude is to be given to the physician. A typical pronouncement is "the doctor's primary duty is to do what is best for the patient. Any conflict between this duty and that of a frightening disclosure ordinarily should be resolved in favor of the primary duty." *Nishi v. Hartwell*, 473 P.2d 116, p. 119.

conflict between the two models of moral responsibility developed in chapter two. Patients' rights and physicians' professional judgments compete in the courts' deliberations.

Contemporary writings in medical ethics on the purposes of informed consent requirements suffer the same problem.[50] One widely shared view is that the primary purpose of informed consent is the protection of autonomy. This description presupposes the dominance of the autonomy model of professional responsibility. However, other purposes of informed consent requirements have also been promoted, in particular the prevention of injury to patients. Informing patients of treatment increases patient cooperation and recovery and presumably avoids those treatments patients consider unjustifiably risky. This second candidate for a primary purpose conforms to the canons of the beneficence model.

There is no *a priori* inconsistency between the dual purposes of protecting autonomy and protecting from harm. But if we believe there is no deep tension between these ideals, we are indulging in the same pattern of wishful thinking reflected in *Salgo*. A direct conflict between full disclosure and physician discretion is inescapable in many interchanges between physician and patient. One's view as to which of these is the *primary* objective of informed consent requirements has decisive implications for several major issues about informed decisionmaking—most prominently for issues about what types and how much information ought to be disclosed if a patient might autonomously reject a physician's compelling medical recommendations and thereby cause injury through his or her autonomous choice.

Patients and physicians, no less than courts, cannot escape a struggle with the dual vision of human nature as at once autonomous and responsible, but needing the same comfort a child does when reduced in decisional capacity by the throes of worry, illness, or injury. The pattern of this problem is everywhere present in medicine, as reflected in circumstances where patients are at once socially functional but mentally ill, partially insistent and partially yielding, partially resistant and partially malleable, depressed but mentally alert, hostile and yet capitulating. The same pattern is also apparent in empirical studies of the quality of decisionmaking by patients: Studies indicate that although *some* patients carefully weigh risks and benefits (among other considerations) when making their decisions about proposed treatments, most follow either their own predispositions or a physician's recommendations, usually without a careful assessment of available information.[51]

---

[50]Several basic functions, purposes, or objectives of informed consent have been distinguished in the influential article by Alexander Capron cited previously: "Informed Consent in Catastrophic Disease Research and Treatment."

[51]See Meisel and Roth, "What We Do and Do Not Know About Informed Consent." Cf. also Ruth R. Faden and Tom L. Beauchamp, "Decision-making and Informed Consent," *Social Indicators Research* 7 (1980): 313–36; and C. H. Fellner and J. R. Marshall, "Kidney Donors: The Myth of Informed Consent," *American Journal of Psychiatry* 126 (1970): 1245–51.

Clinical experience also suggests that patients exhibit wide variability in their capacities to understand and appreciate information about their diagnoses, treatments, or prognoses. While some patients, like Mr. Berkey, seem capable of grasping the particular details of a diagnostic or therapeutic procedure, other patients are excessively nervous, anxious, or distracted—e.g., the older patient who is worried about the word "cancer" and its many meanings, or the adolescent patient with cancer who is obsessed with possible hair loss caused by chemotherapy. Such patients may not, at first, be capable of dealing with information about their diagnosis and treatment. The two visions of the patient's ability to make medical decisions that Katz has identified are also entrenched in the two models of moral responsibility, focused as both are on the problem of decisionmaking responsibility.

WHO SHOULD DECIDE?

Who, then, should decide—the patient or the physician? Who would be so bold as to answer this question with confident finality? Any answer would shipwreck on an infinity of qualifications and in the end would fail to provide more than general guidelines. There is no single or final answer to the question "Who should decide?" because there is no single or final solution to the larger conflict between the two models of moral responsibility. Every rational person wants decisional authority over his or her fate, but who has not known how quickly the contradictory desire to yield to professional authority manifests itself in the face of illness? Everyone wants respect, but like all fundamental moral principles, "respect for persons" can be applied in innumerable ways. One patient may be respected by demanding that he or she resist a desire to capitulate, while another may be respected by lifting the burden of decision from a wearied and tortured soul in need of rest. There can be no single, general answer, substantive or procedural, to the utterly unanswerable and all too general question, "Who should decide?" What can be hoped for instead are physicians well prepared to grapple with the question in light of the moral demands of the beneficence and autonomy models. (This conclusion must not be taken to imply either that in the final analysis the burden of decision rests with the physician or that specific criteria for appropriate decisionmakers can never be adduced for specific contexts. Both assumptions are clearly false.)

General policies that define the physician's responsibilities in the management of information through only one model will inevitably fail. To follow the autonomy model and emphasize only the patient's right to information overlooks clinical realities. Some patients simply are not prepared to hear the physician. Some might be harmed by too much information or poorly timed disclosures, while illness, disease, and catastrophic accidents might have a significant impact on some patients' capacities to decide. To emphasize the beneficence model exclusively is an equally flawed strategy. It can be used to so overemphasize the impact of illness, pain, suffering, and debility that no patient could qualify as autonomous; and it also fails to appreciate the variety of contexts in which physicians manage information—including, for example, genetic counseling or screening for hypertension.

If both models are accepted as the basis of the physician's responsibilities in the management of information, the following three guidelines can be justified. First, patients whose decisional capacities are substantially intact (and who qualify as autonomous) should be treated primarily in accordance with the autonomy model and a subjective standard of disclosure of information that emphasizes relatively complete disclosure. Second, patients whose decisional capacities are substantially impaired by such conditions as severe or profound mental retardation, advanced dementia, emergency situations, and the like (and whose autonomy is thus substantially reduced) should be treated primarily in accordance with the beneficence model, with its characteristic emphases on harms, goods, and the careful monitoring of information. These two guidelines are not together adequate for the full range of patients because many patients are borderline— not substantially autonomous, yet not substantially reduced in autonomy. The effective management of information can itself play a role in the process of overcoming impairments, such as those caused by temporary fear, mild depression, and anxiety. The approach to disclosure with such patients necessarily is directed by a third guideline that involves discretion in the use of both models. The impairment such patients suffer renders the autonomy model inapplicable, but psychological needs for information may nonetheless be present, and effective communication with such patients may be a crucial element in the recovery process.

Many virtues discussed in previous chapters play an essential role in shaping the physician's management of medical information. For example, the virtue of compassion reminds the physician that some of the information may be unpleasant, disturbing, or even frightening, while prudence plays a role in directing the sequence and timing of disclosure so that patients can absorb information in a meaningful way. Patience, too, is of critical importance, especially when dealing with compromised patients. Finally, Osler's *aequanimitas* reminds the physician that "bodily virtues" (whether to sit or stand at the patient's bedside and whether he or she touches the patient and looks at the patient directly) and "mental virtues" (the tone of voice and the balanced exercise of authority) are significant aspects of the physician's moral responsibilities in the effective communication of medical information.

These virtues jointly encourage the virtue of respectfulness. From the fact that a patient may be confused, frightened, or impaired and may have lost the capacity for autonomous decisionmaking, it does not follow that he or she no longer is owed the respect that all of us command. The virtue of respectfulness nowhere applies more insistently than in the management of medical information.

EXTENSIONS AND CONCLUSIONS

We began this chapter with *Berkey v. Anderson,* which served as an introduction to the legal history of informed consent. That history raises, but insufficiently explores, questions about what a physician ought to discuss with a patient in the process of making decisions. While a flood of malpractice cases such as *Berkey* has haunted courts and physicians in recent years, these cases have not, in our experience, profoundly altered medical practice. They have served principally to increase the volume of words in physician disclosures, as well as to increase recorded documentation of disclosure. Most legal pronouncements do not even encourage dialogue, let alone meaningful communication, between patients and physicians.

Nevertheless, if serious dialogue and communication between physician and patient were institutionalized in accordance with the *moral* analyses and arguments set out in this chapter, medical practice might be profoundly altered. The responsibilities of the physician in the management of medical information would be based in a patient-centered standard of communication. For patients whose decisional capacities are adequately intact, this approach would be understood in terms of the autonomy model and the subjective standard: The patient's values and choices would constitute the perspective from which the harms and goods of disclosure should be assessed. For patients whose decisional capacities are seriously impaired, or even absent, the approach would be understood in terms of the beneficence model and the reasonable person standard of disclosure: Medicine's objective values and the (objective) reasonable person would provide the perspectives from which the harms and goods of disclosure should be assessed. For patients whose decisional capacities are basically intact yet whose emotional state may temporarily retard the exercise of sound judgment, the physician must determine the proper balance between the demands of the autonomy model and those of the beneficence model. In reaching this conclusion, we are not rejecting the professional practice standard as a legally appropriate standard in (at least some) malpractice cases. However, we do mean to reject it as a *morally* appropriate standard of disclosure in clinical practice because of the potentially cavalier attitudes toward the patient permitted by such a standard.

Some courts have given indecisive hints in the direction of our conclusions. For example, some have suggested that a physician must render not only an accurate, comprehensible, and sufficiently comprehensive judgment as to the nature, risks, and consequences of a procedure, but also ought to discuss whether the course of treatment should be undertaken at all. The latter question requires a delicate presentation to patients of benefits and risks of particular diagnostic interventions and therapeutic alternatives, without compromising the physician's authority. That is, the physician is asked to render a professional judgment as to the *limits* of what he or she recommends and to discuss those limits realistically with patients.

Much more of an innovative nature needs to be said along these lines than has been said by physicians, courts, and writers in medical ethics. For example, we need to discuss openly how false assurances intended to encourage patients may seriously mislead them; when to disclose to a family information that is judged inappropriate for the patient; how to present information straightforwardly and clearly;[52] and the importance of unhurried, courteous, and properly timed discussions with patients. Disclosure requirements should be discussed in terms not only of what should be said but also what should be asked. The focus should be on the entire communication process, and not simply on disclosure as an obligatory recitation of some stipulated set of facts about risks, benefits, and alternatives. The problem to date with the legal history of disclosure requirements is the near absence of concern about such requirements of communication.

The goal of this chapter has been to elevate our appreciation of the physician's moral responsibilities in the management of information to a greater level of maturity, by arguing against simple resolutions of moral problems surrounding that responsibility. In the case of seriously ill and injured patients who face appreciable risks or frightening choices, the physician's commitment to the patient demands that he or she not abandon the patient to the mere formalities of contemporary legal requirements of informed consent. Let us make no mistake. The physician who deeply cares about the dignity and welfare of patients must operate with and even be trapped between the two models. Both are essential for appropriately dignified and responsible exchanges between physician and patients, and many patients cannot be treated simply in accordance with the demands of one in isolation from the other.

Moreover, we cannot reasonably expect to eliminate the fundamental conflicts arising from the two models and from conflicting legal approaches to the management of medical information. How to address the informational needs of ill, and often compromised, autonomous patients cannot be determined with confident moral generalizations. We can, however, hope to fashion a clearer vision of what it means to treat such patients

---

[52]Variations in the way information is presented to autonomous patients have been shown to significantly influence their seemingly autonomous choices between alternative therapies. See Barbara J. McNeil et al., "On the Elicitation of Preferences for Alternative Therapies," *The New England Journal of Medicine* 306 (27 May 1982): 1259–62.

both professionally and with respect. We can also insist and reinsist on the importance of the virtues and duties of truthfulness and respectfulness in medicine. The importance of discretion in the management of medical information can never excuse the physician from adopting attitudes of self-preoccupation or disrespect.

This general subject is still more difficult to handle than we have admitted in this chapter, as we shall see by addressing the "problem of paternalism"—a problem that unmasks the true depths of our uncertainties about how to care for patients whose capacity for autonomous decisionmaking is substantially affected by their compromised condition.

Chapter 4

Medical Paternalism

Moral problems in the management of medical information were examined in chapter three, but problems of how the demands of the autonomy model are to be balanced against those of the beneficence model plague other areas of clinical practice as well. Problems include whether to employ diagnostic or treatment measures that would benefit the patient but which are resisted by the patient, and whether and to what extent to intervene in the lifestyles of patients in the attempt to change dangerous behaviors such as smoking, excessive alcohol use, and self-destructive dietary habits. If the future health of the patient is at stake, many physicians feel obligated in such circumstances to act on the patient's behalf. They believe that the physician's role is to benefit the patient even if the patient resists.

In the literature on medical ethics, certain problems that arise when physicians act beneficently to protect their patients from harm have been discussed under the rubric of "paternalism" or "medical paternalism." Several competing theories have been developed to show how problems of medical paternalism should be resolved. We examine the most important of these arguments in this chapter. We argue that what seem to be starkly opposed views on the morality of paternalism are often not significantly different. We also argue that the literature on paternalism can easily create a misleading impression of the physician's obligations without revealing what is of importance about medical paternalism. We identify the moral justification of interventions with patients whose autonomy is reduced as the hidden and major problem of medical paternalism. (We then treat this problem in detail in chapter five.) At the same time we argue that some forms of so-called "strong paternalism" can be justified.

A CASE STUDY: A REQUEST
TO DISCONTINUE TREATMENT

In the spring of 1973, a twenty-six-year-old college graduate named Donald Cowart was discharged after three years of military service as a jet pilot.[1] Mr. Cowart had been active in team sports in high school, had performed in rodeos, and was devoted to outdoor activities. He had set his sights on becoming a commercial pilot or lawyer. After his discharge and before moving ahead with his career plans, Mr. Cowart joined his father in a real estate business in East Texas. Two months later he and his father were appraising some rural property about 135 miles east of Dallas. They had unknowingly parked near a leaking propane gas transmission line, and when they returned to start their car, the ignition spark set off a large explosion that engulfed both father and son in flames. After temporary admission to a local hospital, he and his father, both in serious condition, were transferred by ambulance to Parkland Hospital in Dallas. His father died during the two-hour trip to Dallas, a fact Mr. Cowart learned only later.

Mr. Cowart suffered extensive second- and third-degree burns over sixty-eight percent of his body. His ears were largely destroyed, and he was blinded in one eye. Because of gangrene, his fingers were later amputated to the knuckles. His right eye was enucleated (entirely removed) and his left retina was found to be partially detached and the cornea scarred. It was doubtful that sight in that eye could be restored. This eye was surgically sealed shut in order to protect it from infection. Mr. Cowart also underwent skin grafting and daily bathing in a Hubbard tank. He was given pain killers before each tubbing, but not enough to completely relieve the pain of the tubbing and the dressing of his wounds. Mr. Cowart described the pain as excruciating and said he would sometimes pass out when the treatments were completed.

When he was well enough, Mr. Cowart was transferred to a rehabilitation center in Houston, where he was sometimes permitted to refuse the daily tankings that cleaned the burn wounds that remained unhealed. When he became seriously ill from resulting infection, he was transferred to the burn unit at the University of Texas Medical Branch at Galveston, where his recovery was slow and agonizing. He was again given daily tankings, which he found to be extremely painful because of an increased salt content in the water. On one occasion, after the other patient in his room told him the location of the window, he got out of bed intending to jump six stories to his death. However, he was too weak to get to the window and managed only to get out of his bed before his attempt was discovered by his night nurse. After this incident, his roommate was transferred to another room and the tankings were continued.

Throughout these months of treatment in both Dallas and Galveston, Mr. Cowart generally displayed mental alertness—though he recalled some

---

[1]This case is developed from the following sources: Robert B. White and H. Tristram Engelhardt, Jr., "A Demand to Die," *Hastings Center Report* 5 (June 1975): 9–10; a videotape of Donald Cowart's case entitled "Please Let Me Die," University of Texas Medical Branch, Galveston, Department of Psychiatry; and an interview with Donald Cowart at the Kennedy Institute of Ethics in April 1983.

delusional periods very early in his treatment in Dallas. On many occasions he insisted that his treatment be discontinued. Had he been discharged from the hospital, death by infection was inevitable, but he said he intended to take his life, not to allow death to occur by infection. Mr. Cowart's physical condition prevented his leaving the hospital on his own; his discharge required the cooperation of his physicians. As was the case in Dallas, his request to stop treatment was not acted upon by his physicians in Galveston, and the daily baths continued. However, he refused to permit skin grafts to be performed, and this refusal was accepted by his physician, although reluctantly.

A psychiatrist at the University of Texas Medical Branch, Dr. Robert B. White, was consulted to ascertain the legal competence of Mr. Cowart. If the patient were declared mentally incompetent, a legal guardian could be appointed to control permission for further treatment; otherwise, if declared mentally competent, the patient would presumably be as free as any other patient to make decisions regarding the course of his treatment. The results of Dr. White's examination proved surprising to some physicians. He found the patient to be informed, coherent, logical in his reasoning, and rational—thus mentally competent. Nonetheless, Dr. White thought Mr. Cowart's request for release was premature and ill-considered in light of medical improvements that might be achieved in upcoming months. He saw the decision as precipitous, but not as uninformed or nonautonomous. He therefore tried to convince Mr. Cowart to accept further treatment. Mr. Cowart was adamant, however, in his decision to refuse treatment and to die. He insisted that he had the right to control his fate. When he later learned that his refusal to have the skin grafts performed was lengthening the time during which he would suffer the pain of his burn wounds and that this treatment would allow him to shorten his hospital stay, he consented to them. He eventually was discharged and returned to his home in East Texas.

Mr. Cowart's case raises enormously important questions about physician control and the autonomy of patients—questions that are continuous with our discussions in previous chapters of the autonomy model and the beneficence model. Which perspective should determine the patient's best interests—medicine's or the patient's? To what extent should a patient have his or her wishes set aside in light of the physician's judgments about the best that medicine has to offer? To be sure, Mr. Cowart's attending physicians may have known all along what was in his long-range interest; after all, he did survive, and he gained a new perspective on his opportunities and learned to take care of himself. This outcome, however, does not show a complete triumph for the beneficence model in circumstances of unauthorized interventions. Mr. Cowart insisted that he alone had the right to decide whether the treatment was worth the effort, and he had been judged competent by a psychiatrist. He was acutely aware that he would never be able to live the life he once knew, and he was appalled at the failure of those charged with his case to protect what he regarded as his civil liberties. This clash between the beneficent physician and autonomous patient forms the core of the problem of medical paternalism.

WHAT IS PATERNALISM?

The Scope of Paternalism

Paternalism seems to be pervasively accepted in modern society. Examples in medicine include suicide intervention when patients are resistant, resuscitating patients who have requested no further resuscitative efforts, controlling information, various strategies of concealment in psychotherapy, ordering blood transfusions when patients have refused them, forcible invasion of the body through surgery, and small lies or deceptions intended to encourage patients. It has been argued by some that such examples unmask the essentially paternalistic character of patient-physician interactions. Patients are commonly so ill and their judgments or voluntary abilities so significantly affected that they are incapable of grasping important information about their cases. Thus, they are frequently in no position to reach carefully reasoned decisions about medical treatment. Illness, injury, depression, fear, the threat of death, as well as diagnostic and treatment measures can overwhelm patients, rendering them doubtfully able to ascertain their best interests. Every increase in the impact of illness, ignorance, and medical interventions can correlatively enhance the patient's dependence on a physician, leading some critics to assert that hospitals and the medical profession are paternalistic institutions.

This orientation is a prominent theme in the history of medical ethics. In one Hippocratic text cited previously *(On Decorum)*, the physician is enjoined to conceal from the patient "most things." One of the most emphatic expressions of this view in modern medical ethics is found in the first Code of Ethics of the American Medical Association:

> The obedience of a patient to the prescriptions of his physician should be prompt and implicit. He should never permit his own crude opinions as to their fitness, to influence his attention to them. A failure in one particular may render an otherwise judicious treatment dangerous, and even fatal. This remark is equally applicable to diet, drink, and exercise. As patients become convalescent they are very apt to suppose that the rules prescribed for them may be disregarded, and the consequence but too often, is a relapse.[2]

---

[2]American Medical Association, "Code of Medical Ethics," in *Proceedings of the National Medical Convention, 1846–1847* (Chicago: American Medical Association, 1847), as reprinted in Stanley Reiser et al., *Ethics in Medicine* (Cambridge: MIT Press, 1977), p. 30.

The logic of this position is clear. Acting in the best interests of the patient as understood from the perspective of medicine is the primary obligation of the physician; no significant place, therefore, is given to the demands of the autonomy model.

Some recent writers (represented by Soule as well as Loftus and Fries in the previous chapter) support paternalism by arguing that deference to an autonomy model in medicine can be dangerous to a patient's health and can lead to questionable clinical practices that compromise sound medical judgment.[3] They prefer to understand the patient's best interests from the perspective of the beneficence model: "The doctor is bound in his duty to his patient to do whatever is best for his patient and to avoid doing him harm. In discussing his patient's condition, the doctor realizes that there are some circumstances when he cannot, for the patient's own good, tell him the 'whole truth'."[4] This author, Dr. Charles C. Lund, argues that doing as little harm as possible is the *primary* obligation of the physician and that strict control of sensitive information is essential for proper treatment.

On the other hand, the paternalism of the medical profession has come under recent attack, especially by defenders of the autonomy model. They argue that cases like that of Donald Cowart involve an authoritarian exercise of medical control over the life of an autonomous, nonconsenting patient. Physicians have themselves increasingly criticized authoritarianism in their profession. The Judicial Council of the American Medical Association, for example, has said that "social policy does not accept the paternalistic view that physicians may sometimes not divulge information to patients."[5]

The Definition of Paternalism

But what is this paternalism now under such intense discussion? The word "paternalism" traditionally has been used to refer to practices of treating individuals as a father treats his children. As applied to physicians, this analogy turns on two features of the paternal role: (1) the father's

---

[3]In addition to Loftus and Fries, cf. Ronald L. Katz, "Informed Consent: Is It Bad Medicine?" *Western Journal of Medicine* 126 (May 1977): 426–28; Franz Ingelfinger, "Arrogance," *New England Journal of Medicine* 303 (25 December 1980): 1507–11; B. M. Patten and W. Stump, "Death Related to Informed Consent," *Texas Medicine* 74 (December 1978): 49–50; and Steven R. Kaplan et al., "Neglected Aspects of Informed Consent," *New England Journal of Medicine* 296 (12 May 1977): 1127. The Hippocratic influence in creating these views is harshly criticized in Robert M. Veatch, "The Hippocratic Ethic: Consequentialism, Individualism, and Paternalism," in *No Rush to Judgment: Essays on Medical Ethics*, ed. D. H. Smith and L. M. Bernstein (Bloomington, Ind.: Poynter Center, Indiana University, 1978), pp. 238–64.

[4]Charles C. Lund, "The Doctor, the Patient, and the Truth," *Annals of Internal Medicine* 24 (1946): 959. A directly conflicting view, from the patient's perspective, is found in Roger Carus, "Motor Neurone Disease: A Demeaning Illness," *British Medical Journal* 280 (16 February 1980): 455–56.

[5]American Medical Association, Judicial Council, *Current Opinions of the Judicial Council of the American Medical Association* (Chicago: American Medical Association, 1982), p. 26.

beneficence—i.e., acting to protect the best interests of his children; and (2) the father's rightful authority—i.e., his being in an authoritative position that permits making certain decisions for his children that override their wishes or decisions. Similarly, in professional relationships it is assumed that a professional possesses superior knowledge, experience, and skill and has been engaged to further the patient's or client's best interests as the professional understands them in light of that knowledge, experience, and skill. In this respect a professional is sometimes expected to act like a responsible parent, and this is the underlying reason for the choice of the word "paternalism."

"Paternalism" has been used in a more narrow, quasi-technical sense in moral philosophy to refer to practices that restrict or prohibit the autonomous acts of persons without their direct consent. The justification for such actions is either the prevention of some harm these individuals might otherwise cause to themselves or the production of some good for them that they would not otherwise secure. This justification is generally incorporated into the formal definition of paternalism. Accordingly, the following definition of "paternalism" is appropriate: *Paternalism is (1) the intentional limitation of the autonomy of one person by another (2) where the person who limits autonomy appeals exclusively to grounds of beneficence for the person whose autonomy is limited.* The essence of paternalism, then, is an overriding of the principle of respect for autonomy on grounds of the principle of beneficence.[6] While we frequently interfere with an individual's actions in order to protect or promote the welfare of third parties, in paternalistic interferences the goal is solely to protect *that individual's* interests, not the interests of third parties.

It is crucial that the person's *autonomy* is limited. It is not paternalistic, for example, to put an unconscious injured person in an ambulance and send him or her to the emergency room.[7] As applied to the case of Donald Cowart, refusal to release him from the hospital is paternalistic under our definition if it intentionally restricts his autonomy and is performed for his good rather than for the good of others. Some reviewers of Mr. Cowart's case have raised questions about whether he was autonomous during the

[6]This way of depicting the problem of paternalism was perhaps first mentioned by Immanuel Kant, in *On the Old Saw: That May Be Right in Theory But It Won't Work in Practice*, trans. E. B. Ashton (Philadelphia: University of Pennsylvania Press, 1974), pp. 290–291. This framework is developed in systematic detail for medical ethics in Tom L. Beauchamp and James F. Childress, *Principles of Biomedical Ethics* (New York: Oxford University Press, 1979), Chapter 5, and in Robert M. Veatch, *A Theory of Medical Ethics* (New York: Basic Books, 1982), p. 195ff. Not everyone agrees, however, that paternalism always involves a violation of *autonomy*. See, for example, the weakened conditions in James Childress, *Who Should Decide?: Paternalism in Health Care* (New York: Oxford University Press, 1982), pp. 13 and 237ff., and Charles Culver and Bernard Gert, *Philosophy in Medicine* (New York: Oxford University Press, 1982), pp. 130–45.

[7]This misleading example is offered by John Hodson, "The Principle of Paternalism," *American Philosophical Quarterly* 14 (1977): 62.

early periods of his treatment.[8] *If* he was not, then medical intervention would not be paternalistic under our definition of "paternalism." Of course the actual determination of a person's capacity for making substantially autonomous choices often is difficult, and indeed *is* difficult in the Cowart case. On the continuum of autonomy, no sharp theoretical line can be drawn that suffices to distinguish all cases of the autonomous from the nonautonomous. Nevertheless, the definition of paternalism would be severely weakened if "the limitation of autonomy" were not an essential condition. It is also important in medicine to dwell on the conditions justifying intervention without being crippled by uncertainty over whether a patient is or is not acting autonomously.

This understanding of "paternalism" makes the contours of the *moral* problem of medical paternalism clear: Under what conditions, if any, is it justified for one party to override the autonomy of another through beneficent acts, such as diagnostic or therapeutic interventions, in the latter's interest? As Mr. Cowart's circumstances poignantly reveal, medical paternalism arises because of a conflict between the beneficence and autonomy models. This conflict arises from the beneficence model's understanding of the patient's best interests from a perspective that may differ from the patient's perspective on his or her best interests. Before we can attempt to resolve this clash, we must look more closely at the philosophical foundations of both paternalism and antipaternalism—the philosophical positions that, respectively, defend and criticize paternalism in general.

ANTIPATERNALISM AND PATERNALISM

Antipaternalistic Arguments

John Stuart Mill's *On Liberty* (1859) has generally been regarded as the classic philosophical source of antipaternalism. In this work Mill concludes that only harm caused *to another,* not harm caused by oneself *to oneself,* provides a valid ground of intervention with a person's autonomous choices and actions:

> The only purpose for which power can be rightfully exercised over any member of a civilized community, against his will, is to prevent harm to others. His own good, either physical or moral, is not a sufficient warrant. He cannot rightfully be compelled to do so or forbear because it will be better for him to do so, because it will make him happier, because in the opinion of others, to do so would be unwise, or even right. These are good reasons for remonstrating with him, or reasoning with him or persuading him, or entreating him, but not for compelling him, or visiting him with an evil in case

[8]See Robert A. Burt, *Taking Care of Strangers: The Role of Law in Doctor-Patient Relations* (New York: The Free Press, 1979), Chapter 1.

he do otherwise. To justify that, the conduct from which it is desired to deter him must be calculated to produce evil to someone else. The only part of the conduct of anyone, for which he is amenable to society, is that which concerns others. In the part which merely concerns himself, his independence is, of right, absolute.[9]

Mill thus proposes the "harm principle," as it is now generally called: The only valid principle of interference with an individual's autonomy is to protect a *third party*. Interference to protect an autonomous individual from self-caused harm is paternalism and is strictly prohibited. This argument has served as the historical foundation of antipaternalism.

The following letter from a physician, published in 1980 in the *New England Journal of Medicine*, reflects the general attitude of medical antipaternalism, although the concept of paternalism is never explicitly mentioned:

> To the Editor:
> As one who has had a long, full, rich life of practice, service and fulfillment, whose days are limited by a rapidly growing, highly malignant sarcoma of the peritoneum, whose hours, days, and nights are racked by intractable pain, discomfort, and insomnia, whose mind is often beclouded and disoriented by soporific drugs, and whose body is assaulted by needles and tubes that can have little effect on the prognosis, I urge medical, legal, religious, and social support for a program of voluntary euthanasia with dignity. Prolonging the life of such a patient is cruelty. It indicates a lack of sensitivity to the needs of a dying patient and is an admission of refusal to focus on the subject that the healthy cannot face. Attention from the first breath of life through the last breath is the doctor's work; the last breath is no less important than the first.
> Consent by the patient with a clear understanding of this act, by the patient's immediate family, by the family physician, lawyer, minister, or friend should violate no rules of social conduct. There is no reason for the erratic, painful course of the final events of life to be left to blind nature. Man chooses how to live; let him choose how to die. Let man choose when to depart, where, and under what circumstances the harsh winds that blow over the terminus of life must be subdued.
> Frederick Stenn, M.D.
> Highland Park, IL[10]

Two main lines of philosophical argument have been offered in support of the antipaternalism evident in Mill's and Dr. Stenn's thinking. The first is that even limited paternalistic rules in principle allow widespread limitation of liberty that inevitably leads to serious adverse consequences if paternalistic principles are institutionalized. Those concerned about paternalism in medicine are particularly worried about abuses that may result because

[9]John Stuart Mill, *On Liberty*, ed. Gertrude Himmelfarb (New York: Penguin Books, 1974), pp. 68–69.

[10]Frederick Stenn, "A Plea for Voluntary Euthanasia," *New England Journal of Medicine* 303 (9 October 1980): 891.

of the latitude of judgment granted by paternalism to physicians, especially where the personal biases of physicians may result in distortion and even coercion.[11] Those worries are not simply about such matters as assisted suicide, raised by Dr. Stenn. They also concern the full range of patient-physician interaction.[12]

Consider, for example, the findings of Drs. McNeil, Weichselbaum, and Pauker, discussed in chapter two (pp. 47–48), about how patients view the tradeoffs between quantity and quality of life in the face of a serious disease like cancer of the larynx.[13] They argue that it is not enough to simply present a patient with the quantitative aspects of a prognosis, e.g., percentage of survival after a certain period of time. Instead, the way patients assign values to these quantitative outcomes must also be considered. Not doing so might result in a gap between information that physicians disclose and information that is meaningful and important to the patient. The consequence would be a subtle form of manipulation that is unwarranted from the perspective of the autonomy model: Information of genuine importance for the patient's decision—in light of which the patient might change his or her mind—has been shut off.

Paternalism could provide convenient grounds for many such nondisclosures to patients, including the main reason cited by the physicians whose disclosure practices regarding the drug Dilantin were assessed in chapter three: Patients might become unduly alarmed about such risks and refuse medically indicated medication. It is better (or in the patient's best interests), therefore, to withhold this information. The antipaternalist argues that this and similar examples reveal a typical problem in medicine. Physicians overinterpret their paternalistic privileges in circumstances where their patients desire more information or might disagree with an intervention. As a consequence, insufficient weight is given to the patient's understanding of what might be in his or her best interests. A passage from the report of McNeil et al. is worth repeating because it so aptly pinpoints our current problem: "This study [of laryngeal cancer] has a straightforward message: Patients' attitudes toward morbidity are important and survival is not their only consideration. Such attitudes vary enormously from patient to patient. These results seem to preclude *paternalistic* decisions based on 'my clinical experience with patients who have your disease'."[14]

---

[11]For an assessment of the problem of physician bias, see Alan W. Cross and Larry R. Churchill, "Ethical and Cultural Dimensions of Informed Consent," *Annals of Internal Medicine* 96 (January 1982): 110–13.

[12]For an application to Hippocratic medicine, see Veatch, *A Theory of Medical Ethics*, pp. 149–50, 153.

[13]Barbara McNeil, Ralph Weichselbaum, and Stephen Pauker, "Speech and Survival: Tradeoffs Between Quality and Quantity of Life in Laryngeal Cancer," *New England Journal of Medicine* 305 (22 October 1981): 982–87.

[14]Ibid., 987 (emphasis added).

A second and related reason offered in defense of antipaternalism springs from skepticism that physicians (and other authorities) have the ability to know the best interests of patients and families better than patients and families themselves do. Thus, if patients like Donald Cowart are suffering from the pain of disfiguring burns, antipaternalists argue that others, besides the individual actually suffering from the disease or injury, *cannot* know his or her best interests. Thomas Halper has eloquently opposed paternalistic treatment of elderly patients for this reason: "Though the aged citizen will not invariably perceive his own self-interest, he will do so more often than will public officials or even family members, for only he can appreciate his desires, fears, needs, and perspectives with the unalloyed purity of the insider."[15] As antipaternalists see it, such individuals are generally in a position to ascertain their interests more competently than anyone else. If an elderly, competent patient declares that he or she would want to be resuscitated in the event of cardiac arrest because he or she values prolonged life, then he or she should be resuscitated even if family members might object. Here the logic of the autonomy model prevails: The patient's values and beliefs should be the basis for determining what is in his or her best interests.

These two antipaternalistic arguments indicate that one major source of the difference between the supporters and the opponents of medical paternalism rests on the emphasis that each places on abilities of a patient to determine his or her best interests. We shall be in a better position to appreciate the full complexities of this difference between paternalists and antipaternalists after a more careful assessment of the arguments proposed to support paternalism.

Paternalistic Arguments

"Paternalism" is an umbrella term covering numerous possible positions, and many different views have been defended as appropriate forms of paternalism. A continuum of positions is possible, from extensive support of paternalism to very modest support. H. L. A. Hart's characterization of paternalism at many social levels is representative of one extreme point of view: "Paternalism . . . is a perfectly coherent policy. . . . No doubt if we no longer sympathise with [Mill's] criticism this is due, in part to a general decline in the belief that individuals know their own interests best, and to an

[15]Thomas Halper, "Paternalism and the Elderly," in *Aging and the Elderly: Humanistic Perspectives in Gerontology,* ed. S. Spicker, K. Woodward, David D. van Tassell (Atlantic Highlands, N.J.: Humanities Press, Inc., 1978), p. 323. Several arguments against paternalism in health care are collected in Glenn C. Graber, "On Paternalism and Health Care," in *Contemporary Issues in Biomedical Ethics,* ed. John W. Davis, Barry Hoffmaster, and Sara Shorten (Clifton, N.J.: Humana Press, 1978), pp. 233–44, and in Childress, *Who Should Decide?: Paternalism in Health Care.*

increased awareness of a great range of factors which diminish the significance to be attached to an apparently free choice or to consent."[16] Hart
argues that the multitude of factors inhibiting voluntary behavior renders
paternalism a perfectly acceptable practice.

Applied to medicine, this thesis presupposes that for many patients the
physician is in a better position than the patient to determine what is in that
patient's best interests: The patient's autonomy may be limited in order to
protect against consequences whose full significance he or she may not be
able to appreciate. These include situations of unreasonably high risk (e.g.,
being a subject in high-risk medical experimentation), or of potentially
dangerous and irreversible effects (e.g., the risks of some diagnostic, surgical, and pharmacological interventions). Presumably those who support
this position believe it is justified to prohibit Donald Cowart from carrying
out his wish to be released from the hospital and die, on grounds that this
action is irreversibly harmful, his release from the hospital is unreasonably
risky, and the context therefore is one where his physicians are in a better
position than he to know and promote his best interests.

Many paternalists are as concerned as antipaternalists about the sweep-
ing scope some forms of paternalism might assume—in principle "justifying" an extensive array of limitations of liberty. According to this more
limited perspective, paternalism is justified only if: (1) The evils prevented
from occurring to the person are greater than the evils (if any) caused by
the interference with the person's liberty; and (2) It is universally justified
under relevantly similar circumstances always to treat persons in this
way.[17]

Gerald Dworkin has argued that a limited paternalism should be regarded as a form of "social insurance policy" that fully rational persons
would take out in order to "protect themselves."[18] That is, the principle of
paternalism is justified under conditions that would be unanimously
agreed to by a group of impartial rational agents. Such persons would
know that they might be tempted at times to make decisions that are potentially dangerous and irreversible. They might at other times be driven to do
something they would consider too risky if they could objectively assess the
situation. In still other cases, persons might not sufficiently understand or

[16]H. L. A. Hart, *Law, Liberty, and Morality* (Stanford: Stanford University Press, 1963), pp.
31–33.

[17]See, e.g., Charles Culver and Bernard M. Gert, *Philosophy in Medicine*, Chapters 7–8, esp.
Chapter 8.

[18]Gerald Dworkin, "Paternalism," *Monist* 56 (January 1972): 65. His view on this point is
indebted to Rawls. Many writers have subsequently expressed similar views, usually based on
the claim that rational consent justifies paternalism. These writers include Jeffrie G. Murphy,
"Incompetence and Paternalism," *Archives for Philosophy of Law and Social Philosophy* 60 (1974):
481–82; Rosemary Carter, "Justifying Paternalism," *Canadian Journal of Philosophy* 7 (1977):
133–45; and John D. Hodson, "The Principle of Paternalism," *American Philosophical Quarterly*
14 (1977): 65ff.

appreciate the dangers of their conduct, or might distort information about their case. For example, a seriously injured and intoxicated patient, brought to the emergency room following an automobile accident, might physically resist attempts to assess the gravity of what appers to the physician to be serious trauma to the head and major internal organs. To respect such a patient's "refusal" of further diagnostic work-up and admission to the hospital for observation might result in grave risks to the patient, risks the patient cannot appreciate in his or her intoxicated state. Instead of informing persons of the facts and attempting to obtain consent from the patient, which may not be possible, Dworkin and others have concluded that rational agents would voluntarily agree to a limited grant of power to others for paternalistic intervention.[19] Hence, the physician might be justified in working up the patient and treating his injuries, even if doing so involved restraining the patient and forcing medical interventions.

We have found so far that medical paternalists agree that the perspective of medicine can sometimes be legitimately substituted for the patient's perspective. Paternalism thus reflects a reliance on the beneficence model. Not all paternalists, however, go as far as H. L. A. Hart in endorsing a wide-reaching paternalism. Instead, they focus on a limited range of cases in which the patient's ability to make decisions is impaired.

STRONG AND WEAK PATERNALISM

A critical element in the controversy between antipaternalists and paternalists is the *quality* of decisionmaking by patients—in particular the extent to which it is autonomous. Antipaternalists tend to envision and emphasize autonomous choices. They do not regard even serious illness as always mentally incapacitating. Therefore, they tend to view such patients as substantially autonomous and to consider the issues of paternalism from the perspective of the autonomy model. Paternalists, by contrast, tend to envision and emphasize patients who are compromised in their ability to make autonomous choices, i.e., the patient who suffers from temporary depression, fear based on misperception, deep ambivalence, and the like. Paternalists, however, tend to disagree among themselves as to the actual conditions of valid intervention. This leads to an important distinction— widely used, although we shall later question it—between a form of paternalism that intervenes to control only substantially nonautonomous behaviors and a form that controls both these and substantially autonomous behaviors. The former is referred to as weak paternalism; the latter is referred to as strong paternalism.

[19]Dworkin's views are applied specifically to the patient-physician context in Frank H. Marsh, "An Ethical Approach to Paternalism in the Physician-Patient Relationship," *Ethics in Science and Medicine* 4 (1977): 135–38.

Strong paternalism invokes a right to override or prevent autonomous as well as nonautonomous actions of individuals when these actions significantly affect only the individuals themselves. For example, the strong paternalist would presumably intervene to prevent an autonomous suicide and would generally favor a continuation of medical treatment for Donald Cowart. The *legality* of strong medical paternalism has often been tested by cases similar to Mr. Cowart's. In Anglo-American law, the fact that an individual is acting against what most would consider to be his or her best interests does not warrant restriction of his or her autonomy rights—unless the ability to reach an informed decision is seriously impaired. (As we saw in chapters two and three, however, this position is generally tempered by a recognition of the paternalistic need for discretion in releasing information to patients.)

Weak paternalism, by contrast, has been more frequently embraced both in law and moral philosophy. It holds that an individual's self-regarding conduct can be restricted only if it is substantially nonautonomous. If a patient is, for example, psychotic, deeply depressed, in painful labor while in the midst of a delivery requiring a Caesarian section, or suffering from a severe blow to the head, there is good cause to believe that the person's ability to understand is impaired, though perhaps not altogether absent. While he or she might be able to make autonomous decisions regarding selections of food or the time to go to bed, the patient may not be able to process the information necessary to make major medical decisions.

Weak paternalism is predicated on some conception of *compromised* ability: A dysfunctional incompetence or encumbrance is systematically required. The following statement by James Childress expresses this weak paternalism:

> [Paternalism] can be justified under some conditions. For example, paternalistic interventions with regard to children are often justified because children are incompetent in certain areas and are exposed to risk of harm. This example provides two sorts of justification often given for paternalistic interventions: (1) the patient's defects, encumbrances, and limitations, and (2) the probability and amount of harm. If the first of these conditions is held to be necessary for justified paternalism, the position is "weak" paternalism.... I am inclined to consider these two conditions as jointly necessary for justified paternalism [but not as sufficient].... The paternalistic decision maker should also show that the harm to be prevented or the benefit to be provided really outweighs the loss of independence and any other benefits the patient seeks in taking the risks in question.[20]

The analogy to the authority of a father from which the term "paternalism" is derived, as Childress points out, is useful for illustrating weak

<hr/>

[20]James F. Childress, *Priorities in Biomedical Ethics* (Philadelphia: The Westminster Press, 1981), pp. 26–27. See also Childress's similar formulation in *Who Should Decide?: Paternalism in Health Care*, p. 102ff. This latter and more general formulation is not specifically directed at *patients*.

paternalism. Children of age ten, for example, are not altogether *non-autonomous*. They commonly exhibit limited autonomy owing to an insufficiently mature capacity for autonomous decisions. In some areas of their lives they may be autonomous—e.g., in their selection of foods—but in others they may not. Children are classified as minors and as legal incompetents for this reason, and their parents are thereby legally empowered to override those of their children's "choices" that spring from immaturity or diminished abilities. Other groups are similarly treated by social regula-tions and customs. For example, many mentally retarded persons are capable of some autonomous decisions, such as whether to seek new employment or to live in the community in supervised housing. Yet these same persons may have severely limited capacities to make autonomous decisions about a complex medical treatment; and thus they might nonautono-mously inflict harm on themselves. Weak paternalism in medicine is the view that in cases in which a person's ability to make autonomous decisions is substantially reduced with respect to the medical decision at hand, it is justified to override the person's choices and expressed wishes.

All ethical theories hold that it would be unjustified to allow persons to die or suffer serious injury through decisions that are nonautonomous or questionably autonomous. To permit the seriously depressed dialysis patient, the overly frightened stroke victim, or the seriously disoriented elderly patient to go without protection would be callous and uncaring. Our uniform sympathy toward this viewpoint no doubt accounts for the broad support now enjoyed by weak paternalism. On the other hand, an intervention in the lives of such individuals is justified by the weak paternalist's standard *only if there is questionable autonomy*, and not alone because their actions are dangerous or unreasonable. The argument in medical ethics literature about the defensibility of weak medical paternalism thus turns crucially on questions about the patient's level of autonomy. This shift in focus away from paternalism *per se* to reduced autonomy forces us to ask whether there exists the significant difference between weak paternalists and antipaternalists that has commonly been presumed.

WEAK PATERNALISM
AND ANTIPATERNALISM

Defenders of weak paternalism view an undifferentiated antipaternalism as a wholly indefensible doctrine, for it seems to prohibit all forms of beneficent treatment. Who would not compel medical protections for the defenseless leukemic child, the severely mentally retarded individual, the confused and frightened cardiac patient, the hope-exhausted and chronically depressed dialysis patient, and Donald Cowart when he first arrived at Parkland Hospital—protesting his admission all the while? The beneficence model clearly generates obligations to provide necessary care to such patients; any "violation" of the dictates of the autonomy model seems trivial.

Thus, the weak paternalist has, at first glance, every advantage over the antipaternalist. The interventions the weak paternalist defends are clearly justified, while antipaternalism seems locked into a condemnation of them as unwarranted interferences with autonomy. The antipaternalist seems to be the uncompromising devotee of the autonomy model. At the same time, because weak paternalists admit that not all patients are substantially reduced in their ability to make autonomous decisions, they can agree with all the arguments in defense of autonomy that antipaternalists marshal against strong paternalism. Weak paternalism even provides a compromise that prevents one model from overriding the other: It holds that the beneficence model applies only if the patient is substantially reduced in his or her autonomy, while the autonomy model applies in all other cases.

Resolving disputes among paternalists and antipaternalists in favor of weak paternalism—the most popular form of paternalism in medical ethics literature—raises an intriguing question: In light of the precise definition of paternalism, does weak paternalism qualify as *paternalism?* That definition, we recall, requires that paternalism protect an individual from harm or secure a good through limitation of the individual's *autonomy.* In instances of weak paternalism, however, *there is no substantial autonomy to be restricted,* because the decision or action of the patient interfered with is not the patient's own; it is not substantially autonomous. Weak paternalism cannot limit autonomy if it is already substantially limited or absent.[21]

This matter is of immense importance. If the underlying justification for a so-called weak paternalistic intervention is to protect a person from harmful consequences that are *not of his or her making,* then the antipaternalist will not contest that the intervention is justified, and in fact will in no respect disagree. Weak paternalism thus no longer seems distinguishable from antipaternalism,[22] despite a deep assumption to the contrary in the literature on paternalism. This argument may be summarized as fol-

[21]For example, in the widely discussed *Saikewicz* case, involving a severely retarded man ill with leukemia and unable to make medical decisions, the court invoked the legal doctrine of *parens patriae* (the state acting as surrogate parent) in discussing what the state must do to "protect the 'best interests' of the incompetent person." If this form of intervention with incompetents were taken to express paternalism, this usage would render the term "paternalism" so broad as to encompass guardianship—an unsurprising conflation in a legal context, but disastrous for clear philosophical thinking. See *Superintendent of Belchertown v. Saikewicz*, Mass., 370 N.E. 2d 417, p. 427.

[22]As Joel Feinberg noted early in the history of these discussions: "Neither should we expect antipaternalistic individualism to deny protection to a person from his own nonvoluntary choices, for insofar as the choices are not voluntary they are just as alien to him as the choices of someone else." "Legal Paternalism," *The Canadian Journal of Philosophy* 1 (September 1971): 112. This paper is reworked in *Social Philosophy* (Englewood Cliffs, N.J.: Prentice-Hall, 1973); see p. 48. Feinberg's warning has unfortunately been ignored in the subsequent literature.

lows. Both weak paternalism and antipaternalism *agree* on the following two points:

(a)   The justifiability of interference to protect the patient from nonautonomously produced harm; and

(b)   The unjustifiability of interference to protect the patient from autonomously produced harm.

Weak paternalism is thus *not* a form of paternalism that can be distinguished in any interesting respect from antipaternalism.

According to our argument, it only clouds the issue to speak, as does H. Tristram Engelhardt, Jr., of "a paternalism required because of the intrusions of a disease" when a patient's autonomy is overwhelmed by the ravages of disease. Engelhardt maintains that "the more the patient is overwhelmed by the disease process . . . the easier it is to justify a physician's paternalism."[23] If the argument we have advanced is correct, this view is conceptually (though perhaps not morally) misleading. It would better serve clarity to say that the more a disease reduces autonomy the easier it is to justify a *non*paternalistic intervention, or—as we would prefer to say—to justify an intervention *simpliciter.* If a legal guardian overrules an incompetent patient's frightened objection to a needle stick to draw blood for diagnostic testing, the guardian does refuse to accept the patient's "decision," but the reason for authorizing the measure is not paternalistic in any strict sense because *the patient's "decision" is seriously compromised in degree of autonomy.* In such circumstances, the guardian who acts in the patient's best interests intervenes forcibly but not paternalistically.[24]

The problem of suicide intervention provides a useful example to test the thesis that there is no important theoretical or practical difference between weak paternalism and antipaternalism. Donald Cowart had indicated to his physician that he intended to commit suicide after being released from the hospital—a familiar reaction and projection in such dire circumstances. Did the circumstances of his injury and the therapeutic maneuvers that were undertaken cause Mr. Cowart's reaction? Or has he made an autonomous choice? How are we to assess the reasons for and causes of his convictions? Glanville Williams' account of our obligations to persons such as Mr. Cowart provides an interesting perspective on this problem:

> If one suddenly comes upon another person attempting suicide, the natural and humane thing to do is to try to stop him, for the purpose of ascertaining

[23]H. Tristram Engelhardt, Jr., "Rights and Responsibilities of Patients and Physicians," in *Medical Treatment of the Dying,* ed. Michael D. Bayles and Dallas M. High (Cambridge, Mass.: Schenkman Publishing Co., 1978), pp. 18–19. A similar analysis for pediatric patients is found in Norman Fost, "Ethical Problems in Pediatrics," *Current Problems in Pediatrics* 6 (October 1976): 4.

[24]We here reach the opposite conclusion from Charles Culver and Bernard Gert, *Philosophy in Medicine,* p. 60.

the cause of his distress and attempting to remedy it, or else of attempting moral dissuasion if it seems that the act of suicide shows lack of consideration for others, or else again for the purpose of trying to persuade him to accept psychiatric help if this seems to be called for. . . . But nothing longer than a temporary restraint could be defended. I would gravely doubt whether a suicide attempt should be a factor leading to a diagnosis of psychosis or to compulsory admission to a hospital. Psychiatrists are too ready to assume that an attempt to commit suicide is the act of a mentally sick person.[25]

Other psychiatrists do not agree with Williams, relying instead upon the thesis that most suicidal individuals are mentally ill or at least seriously disturbed and therefore incapable of autonomous action. Notoriously, the suicidal patient is often under the strain of a temporary crisis, affected by drugs or alcohol, and beset with considerable ambivalence. Many psychiatric and legal authorities maintain that suicide attempts are almost always the result of maladaptive attitudes that require therapeutic attention going beyond temporary intervention and that those who attempt suicide are not in a position to act in a substantially autonomous manner because they are immature, ignorant, or unduly pressured. The underlying conviction is that the suicidal person suffers from a disease or irrational drive toward self-destruction and is, therefore, nonautonomously attempting to end his or her life. Hence, the business of medicine or behavioral therapy is to remedy the malady and, if possible, to prevent the patient from engaging in self-destructive behaviors in the future.

At present, no available theory adequately explains the motivation to suicide, and we must not try to arbitrate these complicated controversies here. The important point is that weak paternalists and antipaternalists need not dispute over how to handle such cases, for both agree that if suicidal actions of this description are substantially nonautonomous, they generally *should be prevented;* and if they are autonomous, it is generally *unjustifiable to intervene.* Thus, if agreement can be reached about the assessment of Mr. Cowart's mental state and about whether his request to be released from the hospital is or is not substantially nonautonomous, there is no dispute over "paternalism" that would prevent agreement about how to respond.

Let us test this hypothesis further. One of the most plausible cases used to defend weak paternalism has been reported by Mark Siegler and Ann Dudley Goldblatt:

> A young man with a high fever, headache, and stiff neck appeared at the emergency room and gave permission for a spinal fluid examination, which the physician had ordered to test for meningitis. The lumbar puncture confirmed a diagnosis of bacterial (pneumococcal) meningitis, which can be cured easily with antibiotics. But without treatment, it is fatal in three out of four cases, and survivors usually have severe and irreversible physical and

[25]Glanville Williams, "Euthanasia," *Medico-Legal Journal* 41 (1973): 27.

mental impairment. But this patient refused antibiotics when the physician disclosed the diagnosis and prognosis.[26]

Here we have an explicit refusal of lifesaving therapy and a readily available, routine treatment. In their analysis, Siegler and Goldblatt argue that the patient in this case resembles a trauma victim who is profoundly irrational more than an autonomous agent capable of informed consent. They support weak paternalism on the grounds that the patient's capacity for making decisions is severely compromised. However, two features of this analysis are noteworthy. First, Siegler and Goldblatt accept the patient's consent to a spinal fluid examination as valid, but reject the refusal of antibiotics as invalid—an unresolved tension in the analysis. Second, their analysis does not deviate in any significant respect from the framework we have suggested: A medical intervention over the "objection" of the patient can on occasion be justified if the patient is substantially nonautonomous, in which case there is substantially no autonomy to be limited. The antipaternalist would accept the conclusion reached by Siegler and Goldblatt, under their description of the patient's mental status.

The result of our inquiry into the alleged distinction between weak paternalism and antipaternalism in medical ethics literature has been to show that the distinction is untenable—or at least not as firm and clear as might at first appear. Both antipaternalism and weak paternalism agree that it is not warranted for physicians to interfere with the autonomous decisions of patients. When the presuppositions of antipaternalism are probed carefully, it turns out that interventions for patients substantially reduced in autonomy are unobjectionable because no limitation is imposed on autonomy. Thus, antipaternalism and weak paternalism fully agree in their approach to patients in this condition.

One important implication of our inquiry is that *strong* paternalism alone would justify interventions that *override* autonomy. On closer examination, however, the apparent stark difference between strong and weak paternalisms may not be so stark after all. Having challenged the clarity and firmness of the distinction between weak paternalism and antipaternalism, let us therefore consider whether similar considerations vitiate the distinction between strong paternalism and weak paternalism (and hence, because weak paternalism does not differ from antipaternalism, the distinction between strong paternalism and antipaternalism).

---

[26]Mark Siegler and Ann Dudley Goldblatt, "Clinical Intuition: A Procedure for Balancing the Rights of Patients and the Responsibilities of Physicians," in *The Law-Medicine Relation: A Philosophical Exploration*, ed. Stuart F. Spicker, J. M. Healey, Jr., and H. Tristram Engelhardt, Jr. (Boston: D. Reidel Publishing Co., 1981), p. 11.

STRONG AND WEAK PATERNALISM
RECONSIDERED

We again start out inquiry with Mr. Cowart's case. Both the weak paternalist and the antipaternalist—let us imagine—agree with Mr. Cowart's psychiatrist that he is substantially autonomous. The strong paternalist presumably would intervene to continue to treat him, invoking the beneficence model, while the antipaternalist and weak paternalist would resist further intervention, on grounds of the autonomy model. This seems the logical outcome of the theoretical commitments in each case.

A close examination of the writings of those inclined toward what is commonly classified as strong paternalism suggests, however, that defenders of the case for intervention will not, without protest, accept the psychiatrist's assessment of the patient's condition and will not agree that Mr. Cowart is substantially autonomous. Mr. Cowart's "paternalistic" physicians in fact seem not to have accepted this assessment. In justifying their interventions, they and the typical "strong paternalist" refer to factors that influence or fail to influence Mr. Cowart's judgment, such as stress, inexperience, medical ignorance, severe pain, and lack of appreciation of the future. There is rarely a naked appeal to a physician's *paternalistic* interest in the patient's welfare, i.e., one that allows the beneficence model wholly to dominate the autonomy model. Instead, that interest almost always springs from an assumption that a patient like Mr. Cowart has a compromising condition that produces an inability to determine or act in his best interests. Disagreement over the treatment of Mr. Cowart thus springs from different assessments of the patient's condition, rather than from intrinsically different moral viewpoints. *That Mr. Cowart is acting autonomously* is precisely what "strong paternalists" dispute. The interventions they propose, like those of the antipaternalists and weak paternalists, are thus not paternalistic.

A recent article on respect for the autonomy of burn patients can be used to illustrate this analysis. The members of a team in Los Angeles specializing in the treatment of patients like Mr. Cowart have argued that even severely burned patients are indeed alert and competent to make autonomous decisions during the initial hours of hospitalization. The team "aggressively" respects autonomy by supplying patients with information about their condition and prospects and allows the patients to choose between various forms of therapy, including some forms of withholding therapy that portend certain death.[27] This approach has been criticized on grounds that it is doubtful whether burn victims *can autonomously decide* un-

[27]Sharon H. Imbus and Bruce E. Zawacki, "Autonomy for Burn Patients When Survival is Unprecedented," *New England Journal of Medicine* 297 (11 August 1977): 308–11.

der the physical and emotional shock characteristic of such patients.[28] In this controversy there is no dispute about the conditions of valid *autonomy* limitation. The only substantial disagreement crystallizes over assessment of the patient's condition, namely, whether such patients are sufficiently autonomous. Strong medical paternalism may therefore be a position with few if any *pure* proponents, and the justifying reasons used by an alleged strong paternalist may turn out to be similar in kind to those used by weak paternalists and antipaternalists. That is, the appeal may in the end be to inordinately powerful psychological or situational factors that render a person substantially nonautonomous.

It must not be supposed, however, that there *cannot* be cases of strong medical paternalism in its pure form. Purely paternalistic grounds may indeed be invoked for an intervention, and sometimes they are in life-threatening circumstances, such as those resembling Mr. Cowart's. Consider, for example, the case of *Satz v. Perlmutter*. Seventy-three-year-old Abe Perlmutter was mortally ill in a hospital, suffering from advanced stages of amyotrophic lateral sclerosis (Lou Gehrig's disease). There is no cure for this disease and normal life expectancy from the point of diagnosis is two years. Mr. Perlmutter could at this advanced stage breathe only with a respirator and was utterly miserable; the prognosis was death in a short period of time. He was capable of making autonomous decisions, and was fully aware of his perilous circumstances. He requested (with the approval of every family member) that the respirator be withdrawn. His physicians refused to do so because he would die as the direct result. Mr. Perlmutter then managed to remove the respirator himself. An alarm sounded and hospital personnel reconnected the respirator, contending that they had an overriding duty to preserve life. While a refusal to *remove* the respirator might be defended on grounds other than paternalism, the reconnection seems a clear case.[29]

If paternalism is the justification in this case, it would appear that the autonomy model has simply been abused under the influence of an unrestrained beneficence model invoked to justify interferences with patients whose autonomy is intact. We believe that even strong advocates of the beneficence model seldom propose intervention with genuinely autonomous patients on purely paternalistic grounds. (They may, of course, intervene on some grounds other than paternalism—e.g., to spare a family grief or to avoid a murder charge.)

Nevertheless, we do not conclude that strong paternalistic interventions are always unjustified, for this thesis is indefensible. Its indefensibility follows from our claim throughout this book that the principle of respect for

[28]The pertinent criticisms are collected in Childress, *Who Should Decide?: Paternalism in Health Care*, pp. 110 and 125, n. 13. See also Eric Cassell, "Autonomy and Ethics in Action," *New England Journal of Medicine* 297 (11 August 1977): 333–34.

[29]*Satz v. Perlmutter*, 362 So.2d 160 (Florida District Court of Appeals, 1978).

autonomy can be overridden by the principle of beneficence. This can occur if the patient is at high risk of illness or injury, the risk of intervention is relatively low, the risk to the patient's future health and well-being from nonintervention or noncompliance is significant, and the claims of autonomy are minimal. For example, consider a patient with an upper respiratory infection that is bacterial in origin. After describing the nature of antibiotics and their common side effects and gaining the patient's consent to the use of antibiotics, the physician may prescribe the particular antibiotic drug he or she believes to be in the patient's best interest, without consulting the patient about alternative antibiotic medications, some of which may have different side effects. Such nondisclosure also occurs frequently in psychiatry, where alternative modes of (noninvasive) therapy are rarely mentioned. One reason is to avoid undermining the patient's trust and confidence in the mode of therapy in use. Again, a physician may strongly recommend hospitalization for observation and testing of patients with possibly serious illnesses without consulting the patients about alternatives. The physician may carefully monitor the information disclosed so that the risks of intervention are minimized to the patient. The patient is not provided extensive information about alternatives that would be difficult to master and could eventuate in a delay in taking the medication or in being hospitalized. If the physician were to open up numerous options to the patient— none of which could eventuate in a choice by the patient of a reduced level of risk—the result might be to act against the best interests of the patient as understood from the perspective of the beneficence model.

Only a wooden use of the autonomy model would require the physician never to manipulate health behaviors in order to obtain compliance. (That one cannot *always* justifiably manipulate health behaviors was the point of our earlier example of laryngeal cancer.) In the instance of the antibiotics prescription, as described above, the patient faces a serious, potentially impairing, and even life-threatening condition. No significant risk is assumed for the patient if the physician determines the drug of choice and makes the decision about how to treat the condition appropriately. In the hospitalization case, the physician is able to gather urgently needed information in a timely and systematic fashion, thus directly benefiting the patient by establishing an adequate data base for future decisions by both patient and physician. Moreover, obtaining further information about the patient's condition involves only the inconvenience of a short stay in the hospital. No significant risk is presented by hospitalization, and no decisions about whether to employ invasive tests or to introduce any significant treatment are seized from the patient.

Consider the following case: A forty-five-year-old woman with recently diagnosed diabetes, which she has not been able to control through diet changes, presents with chest pains. She has a history of serious medical noncompliance, rooted not in resistance but in weakness of will and in a mild fear of doctor's offices and hospitals. An electrocardiogram reveals that she has irregular heart function: atrial flutter and atrial fibrillation. Neither is necessarily an immediate life-threatening condition, but in the presence of uncontrolled diabetes they are cause for serious concern. In order to determine an appropriate course of treatment for the patient, the physician requires more information, which can be best obtained through tests most effectively conducted in the hospital. In addition, the course of treatment involves the use of drugs with complications best managed in a hospital setting. Should the drugs fail to correct the irregular function of her heart, further treatment, such as the induction of electric current to attempt to stop the irregular function, is administered only in a hospital.

In such circumstances a physician would surely be justified in telling the patient that she should be admitted to the hospital without delay and that arrangements for immediate admission have been made. This patient faces significant risk of compromised health, and any risk of hospitalization is minor. The tests to be used are noninvasive and pose minimal risk. Moroever, further testing is essential for a prompt and precise diagnosis of her problem. Finally, her fear of hospitals can be addressed during her initial work-up in the hospital and throughout the course of her stay, and thus minimized as a potential obstacle. Doing so would set the stage for future treatment, which also will most likely involve hospitalization. Suppression of information about the possibility of out-patient management of her condition thus avoids the risks of an incomplete diagnosis and possible noncompliance should hospitalization for treatment be required later. The weight of obligation under the beneficence model clearly is greater than that of the autonomy model and justifies the physician in taking appropriate measures to admit the patient to the hospital.

These arguments and cases suggest a general justification for strong medical paternalism: It can be justified (but will not *always* be justified, depending on the patient and other circumstances) if (1) the risk of nonintervention by the physician or noncompliance by the patient is highly significant, (2) the risk of the medical intervention is minor, and (3) the limitation of autonomy presented by the intervention is a minor limitation. In the paradigm instance of justified strong paternalism, the risk of noncompliance is serious, while diagnostic measures (for example) are low in risk, or even free of risk, and the limitation of autonomy is not of major significance to the patient in the circumstances. The final condition generally implies that no significant values or beliefs of the patient are at stake in the proposed intervention. In the case of Jehovah's Witnesses and blood transfusions, for example, such values and beliefs are at stake. (See chapter two.) Significant values can be used to ascertain whether the limitation of autonomy is of relatively minor or greater importance to the patient. We believe that this approach to the care of patients is already a routine part of medicine, and one that is thoroughly justified if the above three criteria apply.

This argument helps us appreciate why such virtues as steadiness and authority—first developed by Percival and later in the first AMA Code of Ethics and the work of Austin Flint—should be cultivated by physicians. Such virtues aid the physician in managing patient care by keeping an unwavering eye on obligations to promote the patient's best interests. Of course, steadiness and authority can turn to harshness and blind authoritarianism, and for this reason Percival insists that these virtues must be tempered by other virtues such as tenderness to make the paternalism of the physician humane, rather than wooden, cold, or harsh.

A similar view has been reaffirmed in contemporary medicine by the late Franz Ingelfinger, a distinguished physician and editor of the *New England Journal of Medicine*. Based on his personal experience as a cancer patient, Ingelfinger endorses the virtue of arrogance "in the sense of paternalism and dominance" exercised in "beneficial medical care."[30] Arrogance, as a trait of character or habit of the physician, benefits the patient by preventing anxiety about his or her diagnosis, treatment, and prognosis from becoming overwhelming. Like Percival, Ingelfinger is aware of attitudes that could turn arrogance into harsh and inhumane indifference; he warns against counterfeit versions, those in which "insolence, vanity, arbitrariness, and a lack of sympathy" substitute for benefits to the patient: "In other words, a physician can be beneficially arrogant, or he can be destructively arrogant."[31]

An important parallel to our arguments is found in the relationship between lawyers and clients, where lawyers have traditionally been granted truly extraordinary paternalistic powers to override the decisions of clients about legal tactics. In *Nelson v. State,* a court denied a client the right to have his lawyers follow his proposed legal strategy: "Our reasons are that only counsel is competent to make such a decision. . . . One of the surest ways for counsel to lose a lawsuit is to permit his client to run the trial. . . . If such decisions are to be made by the defendant, he is likely to do himself more harm than good."[32]

Extensive paternalism in patient care could be the *practical outcome* for medicine of the theoretical position we have advanced in this chapter, and this result is the natural fear of every lover of autonomy. We therefore must not leave this subject without one final caution regarding the dangers of strong medical paternalism in the "routine part of medicine." Strong paternalism emerges as a problem in medicine because of a conflict of values between physician and patient. "Doctor knows best" is a powerful, however

[30]Franz J. Ingelfinger, "Arrogance," 1510.

[31]Ibid., 1510.

[32]As quoted from "Patients, Clients, and Workers: The Right to Decide," in *Report from the Center for Philosophy and Public Policy* 2 (Fall 1982), ed. Claudia Mills, p. 10.

subtle, motivation to physicians in cases of conflict; they often see capitulation to values held by patients as a sacrifice of professional judgment in deference to a patient's foolish choice. Like a specter hanging over medical practice, paternalism lurks in the very conception of the physician's commitment to the patient. Physicians all too readily reach for a psychiatric consult to justify their point of view in these contexts,[33] and there are infinite dangers in carrying the justification of strong paternalism too far. It has been our intention to *limit* paternalism's role severely, not to signal to physicians that they should always treat patients as their professional wisdom dictates.

Our consideration of the distinction between weak and strong paternalism thus has two results. First, in serious or life-threatening cases where the patient is resisting required treatment, those who appear to be strong paternalists generally turn out to be weak paternalists: They hold that the patient is substantially diminished in autonomy, and this partially justifies the intervention, just as it does in Childress's defense of weak paternalism. The second is that in less serious, more routine cases, which do not necessarily involve only life-saving treatment, a form of strong paternalism is sometimes justifiable. It is legitimate to appeal to the beneficence model as the primary guide for physician conduct because the claims of the beneficence model are compelling, and there are good reasons to believe that the concerns of patient autonomy are minimal. Even in these circumstances, however, one must have reference to *both* models in justifying this approach; that is, one must not simply invoke one model to the complete exclusion of the other.

Unlike confident proclamations delivered in various writings on medical paternalism, there can be no acceptable general solution to this problem of balancing models by opting for one exclusively, any more than there can be such a solution to the problem of conflicting models discussed in chapter two or the problem of conflicting visions of human capacities for decisionmaking discussed in chapter three. There is no comprehensive solution to "the problem of paternalism," because the moral problem is structurally the same as that encountered in chapters one through three: How are we to *weight* considerations of the patient's autonomy against competing considerations of beneficence? In answer to this question, no moral principle and no model of responsibility has a standing trump to play. We cannot determine *a priori* how much weight to give to the principles of respect for autonomy or beneficence in the event of conflict. Instead, the preceding analysis of distinctions between paternalism and

---

[33]See Mark Perl and Earl Shelp, "Psychiatric Consultation Masking Moral Dilemmas in Medicine," *New England Journal of Medicine* 307 (2 September 1982): 618–21. They are concerned that moral problems may be masked as psychiatric problems and that the psychiatrist may inappropriately assume expertise in moral matters.

antipaternalism and between strong and weak paternalism has shown that under certain criteria strong paternalism is justified, and in all too many cases of "strong" and "weak" paternalism, the debate over "justified paternalism" is not a debate about *paternalism* in the strict sense at all, because no interference with a patient who is substantially autonomous is contemplated. *Whether to intervene on behalf of patients with reduced autonomy* is the real problem in these cases; "medical paternalism" is the philosopher's misidentification of the issues they raise for the moral responsibilities of physicians.

CONCLUSION

The problem of medical paternalism should thus be reconceived as a set of problems about determinations of autonomy and competence, eventuating in questions about how to justify diagnostic and therapeutic interventions in cases where a patient is at a level of questionable or reduced autonomy and in need of medical care. We have taken only an initial step toward developing a more comprehensive theory of justified intervention for patients with reduced autonomy. If a comprehensive theory could be developed, we believe the problem of paternalism—as that subject is presently discussed in much of the literature on medical ethics—would largely wither and die.

Much that a physician does, to many a patient's eternal gratitude, is to make the sick feel better. Yet often not much can be done for a patient, and many promising or helpful cures turn into disappointments. The childlike, dependent, and even regressive behavior exhibited by some patients in the presence of physicians—one dimension of the patient's vulnerability—often bespeaks the patient's need for authoritative utterance and a sense of trained and experienced competence, including what Ingelfinger terms "arrogance." The physician, like other professionals with their clients, is expected to recommend and encourage, not merely to offer options. It is therefore understandable that a physician under any measure of influence by the beneficence model might conceive his or her responsibilities paternalistically. This mantle need have nothing to do with rudeness or ignorance; it can be a perfectly justifiable exercise of authority, in a context where persons need help and care.[34] Obviously, it could be generalized beyond medicine, but the further we stray from contexts where people willingly seek and desperately need the help of others, the more implausible and dangerous such use of authority become.

[34]On this theme, see Ingelfinger, "Arrogance," 1509; and Stuart J. Youngner and David L. Jackson, "Commentary: Family Wishes and Patient Autonomy," *The Hastings Center Report* 10 (October 1980): 21–22.

While all rational persons crave some decisional authority over their medical fates, we must all recognize how disease and injury can affect even the most hardy and resistant among us. The physician must face this fragile and unpredictable trait of human behavior daily, without glimpsing the worlds of work, family, and leisure in which the patient, in better times, exudes the normal confidence that attends uninhibited autonomous decisionmaking. We must expect physicians to make occasional mistakes of paternalism, even badly misjudging the actual needs of their patients. Martha Lear's *Heartsounds* gives a penetrating account of the mistakes of a wife and a surgeon in hiding information from her husband about his actual condition and postsurgical complications over a four-year period. Once her husband came to understand how much had been concealed, he assessed his physician's actions as follows: He "may not have told me in order to protect me, . . . and I think that was wrong, but I know he meant well. He didn't understand, though. *None* of you understood: the truth would have been *easier*."[35]

The logic of this chapter develops from the arguments in previous chapters: The beneficence and autonomy models together justify the moral responsibilities of physicians. A patient should not be treated in terms of extremes: neither simply as the instrument of the doctor's professional wisdom and reassuring authority (the beneficence model exclusively), nor simply as the bearer of indefeasible rights to all diagnoses, records, and possible courses of therapy (the autonomy model exclusively). We are left, then, with a pressing problem: How are we to understand the physician's obligations to patients whose autonomy is reduced? This issue has been hidden behind the sometimes furious debates in the literature on medical paternalism about the types and justifications of medical paternalism, and we must subject it to careful analysis in the next chapter. To do so, we must develop clear concepts of reduced autonomy and diminished competence and explain their bearing on the physician's moral responsibilities.

---

[35]Martha W. Lear, *Heartsounds* (New York: Simon and Schuster, 1980), p. 267 (emphasis added).

Chapter 5

Reduced Autonomy
and Diminished Competence

In the previous chapter we saw that most disputes about paternalism have less to do with a "paternalistic principle" than with justifying appropriate interventions for patients with reduced autonomy. When such patients are not able to make autonomous decisions—whether for or against medical care—the weight a physician should give to their choices is uncertain. An ambivalence with the same roots will bedevil us throughout this chapter. In *The Killing of Bonnie Garland,* psychiatrist Willard Gaylin reflects on our contemporary use of the insanity defense in criminal trials. He argues that a sharp tension between the fundamental premise of law and the fundamental premise of psychiatry is at work in these trials: The premise of law is the autonomy of the person; the premise of psychiatry is that the self is a geyser of impulses erupting in various behaviors. The law assesses responsibility and fault; psychiatry seeks to cleanse our vocabulary of such terms.[1] The issues we encounter in this chapter are logically and historically tied to these problems. The concept of reduced autonomy and the related concept of diminished competence emerge from the intersection of law and psychiatry much in the way that insanity defenses engage the two disciplines. At stake is the significance for physicians of judgments of reduced autonomy: What intervention is the physician justified in employing for a patient with such reduced capability?

We approach this question, first, by examining the nature and significance of the continuum of reduced autonomy from mildly reduced autonomy to substantially reduced autonomy. Second, because issues surrounding reduced decisional capacity are addressed in medicine in terms of *competence* and *incompetence,* we provide an analysis of these notions. Third, we analyze some problems in justifying interventions for patients with reduced autonomy and consider some guides for treating such patients. Throughout this inquiry the following three cases are examined.

---

[1]Willard Gaylin, *The Killing of Bonnie Garland: A Question of Justice* (New York: Simon & Schuster, 1982).

THREE CASE STUDIES

A Refusal of an Invasive Diagnostic Procedure

Mrs. Simpson is a seventy-five-year-old woman whose husband died eight years ago. She lives with her daughter and son-in-law and their two teenage children. Mrs. Simpson suffers from arthritis, especially in the elbow and wrist joints. She also has organic brain syndrome and is intermittently confused. When lucid, she can participate in limited daily activities at home, such as helping to prepare meals, doing laundry, and other domestic chores. She is, however, largely home-bound and goes out only in the company of her daughter, son-in-law, or grandchildren, to shop for clothes and to attend church services.

One afternoon Mrs. Simpson is brought by her daughter to the emergency room with a chief complaint of shortness of breath. Physical examination is inconclusive, but radiographic diagnosis reveals a "coin" lesion in Mrs. Simpson's right lung. The radiologist offers a probable diagnosis of cancer and the physician recommends that a bronchoscopy[2] be performed to confirm or rule out the diagnosis of cancer. This procedure is not inherently dangerous and is performed when the patient is sedated. When presented with the request for a bronchoscopy and an explanation of its purpose, Mrs. Simpson says that she does not want a tube stuck down her throat and insists that she is fine. She says that she does not know what all the fuss is about and just wants to go home.

Her daughter, however, says that her mother is confused, is acting out of character, and does not know what she is doing. A psychiatric consult is requested, and a mental-status examination reveals that Mrs. Simpson suffers impairment of short-term memory and is disoriented as to place and time. She is also agitated and distracted. The psychiatrist says that, while Mrs. Simpson might not be declared incompetent for the purposes of all medical decisionmaking, he does not find her refusal to be based on "appropriate reasoning processes." When presented with this information, Mrs. Simpson's daughter insists that the bronchoscopy be performed in order to determine the seriousness of her mother's problem.

Pharmacological Treatment for a Possible Depression

Mrs. Babcock is an eighty-two-year-old woman whose husband died fifteen years ago. Their only child, a son, died at the age of twenty-five. She lives alone in a large urban apartment complex for the elderly and disabled,

---

[2]Bronchoscopy involves placing a tube down the trachea or "windpipe," to examine the interior of the bronchia or branches of the trachea within the lung.

which is part of a planned neighborhood housing development. She is an avid reader.

Six months ago, her only surviving blood kin, a nephew, died. He and his wife and child used to visit her regularly, and she felt particularly close to the nephew. Since his death, his widow has visited Mrs. Babcock only infrequently. Four years earlier, Mrs. Babcock had suffered chronic depression. As a consequence, she failed to maintain proper nutritional habits, became anemic, and suffered significant weight loss. She had been hospitalized at the request of her nephew and had undergone a variety of treatments, including electroshock therapy, which had relieved her depression. After leaving the hospital, she had been placed on a drug regimen of antidepressants, but she stopped this regimen after six months. At that time she felt better and complained about the side effects of the drug, including nausea and grogginess. Since that time she has shown no new signs of depression.

Mrs. Babcock has now come to see her doctor, a second-year resident in family medicine, for problems with sleeping and heart palpitations. After some prodding by her physician, Mrs. Babcock says that she is afraid of dying alone and is worried that because she will have no survivors, she will not receive a proper funeral. In addition, she says that she is concerned about crime in her neighborhood and in her building. She has become so concerned that she leaves her apartment only in the daytime and only to go grocery shopping once a week. She no longer visits her women friends in the apartment building because their problems—which all have to do with living alone and in fear of crime—only recall her own. She also remarks that ten of the elderly residents in her building have died in the last two months, leading her to wonder when her time will come. When her physician suggests that she become more active and perhaps participate in a foster-grandparent program,[3] Mrs. Babcock visibly brightens and says she would enjoy such activity since it would get her out and allow her to enjoy life more.

Her physician discusses her concerns further and promises to obtain information on memorial societies, which will help her to plan for her funeral. He also schedules a home visit in two weeks. At chart rounds at the end of the day,[4] the attending physician suggests that, in light of the patient's history and present condition, the resident consider starting Mrs. Babcock on antidepressants again, to be on the safe side. The resident replies that Mrs. Babcock disliked the drugs she took before, and might resist. The attending physician replies that Mrs. Babcock's problem might be

---

[3]The foster grandparents program is a public program that matches elderly citizens with children, for whom the elderly person becomes a "foster" grandparent.

[4]Chart rounds consist in meetings at which the charts or medical records of patients seen during the day are reviewed by residents and attending (supervisory) physicians.

organically based. If so, she is at risk of becoming depressed and vegetative again, running the additional risk of significant medical problems, including malnutrition and possible suicide. The attending physician recommends strongly that the resident start Mrs. Babcock on an antidepressant drug regimen, even if she dislikes the side effects of the drug.

A Patient Considering Suicide

Mr. Perry is a thirty-six-year-old accountant with a wife and three children, Amy, eight, George, six, and Cathy, three. A scalene lymph node biopsy has shown him to have immunoblastic lymphadenopathy, a uniformly fatal, malignant tumor of the lymph node structures. Consequently, there are no real options for survival open to Mr. Perry, and he has been so informed. Since the lymph node biopsy, he has received maximal radiotherapy, chemotherapy, and immuno-suppressive therapy. Despite these measures, his disease has continued to progress, and he has been made well aware that all surgical and medical measures that hold out the possibility of cure have been exhausted.

Mr. Perry suffers daily from excruciating nerve root pain, which has required the administration of narcotics to the point of significant dependence, perhaps addiction. Higher dosages will not completely free him from pain and might be lethal. Because of spinal cord destruction and bladder dysfunction, he moved into a long-term care facility three months ago. The cost of this institutionalization is rapidly exhausting his family's meager savings. He has accumulated over $6,000 in unpaid and noncompensable health care costs during his illness, which he and his wife must eventually cover. (He has a life insurance policy worth $25,000.) He has no strong religious beliefs, but has been counseled by a minister. His upbringing was Christian. He seems reconciled to his immediate death, perhaps with "dignity," yet death has not been forthcoming.

For some time he has considered suicide, at first fleetingly but, with the onset of his pain, more seriously and consistently. For a brief period after first using narcotics and the relief they brought, he put this notion aside, but with the onset again of the pain he is reconsidering suicide. He says to his physician that suicide may be a humanitarian, altruistic option to end his own and his family's suffering, and to protect their dwindling economic resources. He has discussed these thoughts for several weeks with his physician but has expressed reluctance to ask for the physician's direct assistance to end his life.

One morning he tells his physician that he has procured the means to end his own life, quietly and without manifest detection, embarrassment, or abnormal grief to his family. After several long conversations, the physician understands his determination and his evident willingness to end his life. In these discussions Mr. Perry has reasoned that his death would end his physical pain and anguish and stop the drain on family savings. His physical and emotional reserves, he judges, have collapsed. It would also end his wife's long vigil. Her emotional reserves, he thinks, have been nearly exhausted, an assessment in which the physician concurs. Mr. Perry detects a disturbing ambivalence on his wife's part about his continued existence, although he has not asked her for help in ending his life. Mr. Perry's physician has observed that, on several occasions after visiting her husband, Mrs. Perry sits quietly in the waiting room with their three children, hugging them as she cries. They ask why she is crying, and she is unable to offer an explanation.

Mr. Perry requests that, should he attempt suicide, his physician not interfere. He requests that he not be resuscitated and that a "no code" order[5] be entered into his chart by his physician.

These three cases involve patients whose levels of autonomy are uncertain. Mrs. Simpson's autonomy seems reduced because of an underlying pathology—organic brain syndrome. Mrs. Babcock's autonomy to decide about pharmacological intervention to treat her possible chronic depression is in question; she may already be significantly depressed due to organic disorders and environmental stresses, but she also may not be. Finally, while Mr. Perry seems to have thought through his decision with some care, intense emotion underlies his reflections, complicated by his pain and drug regimen, all of which call his autonomy into question.

It is uncertain how much weight the physician should assign to the decisions of each of these patients, especially where there is ambivalence or behavior that is out of character for the person. Each reduction in the capacity for autonomous choice presents a new challenge. But what is reduced autonomy, and how should physicians care for patients with reduced autonomy?

REDUCED AUTONOMY
IN PATIENTS

The physician, as a rule, must respect the decisions of autonomous patients. However, this rule may not apply if the patient's decisions derive from a lack of knowledge, lack of understanding, or lack of independent judgment. We shall use the term "reduced autonomy" to characterize those instances in which these deficiencies reduce autonomy in the sense discussed in chapter two. Anxiety or depression, as in the case of Mrs. Babcock, might be the source of reduced autonomy, as chronic pain might

[5]A "no code" or "do not resuscitate" order in the chart means that, should the patient's heart or respiratory functions stop, no effort will be made to restore either (or both) function(s).

be in the case of Mr. Perry. Two questions emerge regarding minimally reduced and substantially reduced autonomy—and every form of reduced autonomy in between. What is the significance to the physician of a reduction in patient autonomy? What are the criteria for determining the presence of reduced autonomy? Let us consider each question in this order.

The Significance of Reductions in Autonomy

The extent to which a patient's decisions are autonomous is sometimes difficult to determine, as the three case studies above indicate. Drs. David L. Jackson and Stuart Youngner reached this same conclusion after examining numerous cases of patients' decisions in a medical intensive care unit.[6] In these cases, the patient's life is often at stake if treatment is refused, and these authors properly caution against "superficial preoccupation with issues of patient autonomy and death with dignity."[7] Such preoccupation may lead the physician to act on treatment "decisions" by patients who would be inappropriately described as autonomous; a critically ill patient, they contend, often has "little autonomy." As a consequence, sound clinical judgment might be abandoned in favor of a superficial or simplistic application of the autonomy model.

Jackson and Youngner have identified psychological factors that interfere with what they call "true autonomy."[8] These factors include deep ambivalence about treatment, fear based on misperception, depression, a plea for death with dignity that expresses a "hidden problem," and conflict with the family's perception of a patient's best interests. For example, these authors note that many patients are so ambivalent about their wishes that it is difficult to determine whether a refusal of treatment is the person's autonomous decision. They argue that physicians must neither unquestioningly accept such a refusal nor interpret the patient's behavior exclusively from a perspective intelligible to them as physicians. Instead, the physician should continue treatment, even in the face of objections, until better communication and reduced ambivalence have been established. Only then can "true autonomy" be established—if it can be established at all.

These psychological factors apply to our three cases: Mrs. Babcock's resistance to taking antidepressants might be based as much, if not more, in her depression and fear of death as in her reasoned evaluation of the side effects of the drug. Mr. Perry's request that his suicide attempt not be impeded might be based as much in an emotionally colored concern to end his wife's suffering, and his suffering in the face of her ambivalence, as in a

---

[6]See David L. Jackson and Stuart Youngner, "Patient Autonomy and 'Death with Dignity'," *The New England Journal of Medicine* 301 (23 August 1979): 404–8; and their "Commentary: Family Wishes and Patient Autonomy," *Hastings Center Report* 10 (October 1980): 21–22.

[7]Jackson and Youngner, "Patient Autonomy and 'Death with Dignity'," 407.

[8]Ibid., 408.

reasoned evaluation of his pain, his future possibilities, and his family's future financial stability. We must, of course, not conclude that merely because a patient exhibits anxiety and the like, he or she cannot make a substantially autonomous choice. Nevertheless, because of the ambiguity surrounding these cases, it is uncertain how much moral weight the physician should invest in Mrs. Babcock's resistance or in Mr. Perry's request for a "no code" order (as well as in any "decisions" by patients with reduced autonomy—decisions both against and for medical assistance).

Jackson and Youngner argue that disease and its sequelae can reduce autonomy, but that we must be cautious in reaching such judgments. Reductions in autonomy come in degrees, with differing implications for the physician. While their findings alert us to the *significance* of reductions of patient autonomy, they only hint at factors that should influence physicians in handling the wishes of patients. Let us turn first to factors about patients that properly influence physicians, and then to criteria of reduced autonomy.

Factors that Influence Physicians

Mark Siegler, a physician who writes in medical ethics, has made an important attempt to identify appropriate physician responses to the choices made by patients whose autonomy is reduced.[9] In an examination of the impact of critical illness on patient autonomy, Siegler correctly holds that there are two polar positions on the limits that an autonomous patient may place on diagnostic and therapeutic care once a physician has recommended the care. One position emphasizes (to resort to our categories rather than Siegler's) the autonomy model and demands that treatment not be provided if refused by the autonomous patient.[10] The other polar extreme relies on the beneficence model: An autonomous patient's refusal or other wish may be overridden if the refusal has serious medical consequences, and the patient must not prevent the physician from carrying out his or her responsibilities to treat.[11] Siegler argues, quite reasonably, that both extremes fail to consider "the medically and morally relevant factors

[9]Mark Siegler, "Critical Illness: The Limits of Autonomy," *The Hastings Center Report* 7 (October 1977): 12–15.

[10]Siegler identifies this alternative with the writings of Professor Robert Veatch. This interpretation clearly must be qualified in light of Veatch's views on weak paternalism. See his *A Theory of Medical Ethics* (New York: Basic Books, 1981), Chapter 8.

[11]Siegler identifies this "alternative attitude" with the views expressed by Dr. Eric Cassell in "The Function of Medicine," *The Hastings Center Report* 7 (December 1977): 16–19, esp. 16. See also Cassell's "Autonomy and Ethics in Action," *New England Journal of Medicine* 297 (11 August 1977): 333–334. Siegler unfortunately ignores Cassell's statement (17) that "it does not appear to me to be a truly autonomous act" when the patient refuses under such conditions of illness. Because Veatch (see note 10) limits his views to autonomous agents, the differences between them and the models they represent is imprecisely joined. This is the problem we detected throughout Chapter 4 in most theories of paternalism.

that physicians assess when determining whether to respect the wishes of critically ill patients" because neither extreme adequately appreciates "the particularities of clinical circumstances."[12]

Siegler identifies six factors that legitimately influence the physician's decision about how to handle the wishes of critically ill patients. These factors are the following:

1. *The patient's ability to make (rational) choices about care.* Does the patient have sufficient intellect and rationality to make choices?
2. *The patient's consistency with his or her values.* Are the "choices" made by the patient consistent with his or her values, and are the choices sufficiently independent of (not controlled by) the values of others?
3. *Age.* A more mature patient's refusal in life-threatening circumstances can sometimes be more easily respected than the refusal of much younger persons.
4. *Nature of the illness.* Whether the illness can be diagnosed and what the prognosis is can be significant, especially if complete recovery is possible with appropriate treatment.
5. *The attitudes and values of the physician responsible for the decision.* The physician's moral and religious background, attitudes toward life and death, and the like, have an unavoidable role to play in the physician's choice.
6. *The clinical setting.* When authority is diffused among a health care team, decisions must be reached in ways different from those used in such private settings as the physician's office, a patient's home, or a nursing home.[13]

The first two factors on Siegler's list are the most relevant to our concerns in this chapter. The first factor he characterizes as the patient's capacity to exercise a "degree of discimination and choice." The patient must comprehend and appreciate (in the senses discussed in chapter three) the facts about his or her present condition, the diagnosis, the implications of treatment and nontreatment for the conditions, and the prognoses with and without treatment. The second factor Siegler refers to as the patient's "baseline personality"—the "personality, character, ideas, and beliefs" of the patient. "Baseline personality" refers to normal, consistent behavior of the patient, as well as his or her "commitment, expressed through time," to certain values. This stable personality provides a standard against which the physician can compare the behavior and decisions of the patient; the

---

[12]Siegler, "Critical Illness: The Limits of Autonomy," 13. That Siegler's analysis ultimately depends on the role of "clinical discretion" is clearer in his "Commentary: Does 'Doing Everything' Include CPR?" *The Hastings Center Report* 12 (October 1982): 28–29.

[13]Siegler, "Critical Illness: The Limits of Autonomy," 13–15. We do not wholly endorse Siegler's sixfold list, because there are strong reasons to think that some of these factors—most noticeably #5—ought to be irrelevant to treatment decisions. Imagine, for example, how this criterion might intrude in Mr. Perry's case, with unfortunate paternalistic outcomes. Nonetheless, Siegler does correctly maintain that certain factors that draw together autonomy and beneficence do and ought to influence the physician's decision whether to respect a patient's expressed wishes.

ground of moral responsibility is found in those decisions by a patient that are "consistent with his previous behavior and values."[14] Siegler is insistent, and rightly so, that decisions expressing a patient's stable values are critical to a determination of autonomy.

This idea is sometimes expressed in the literature of medical ethics in terms of the patient's "authenticity" or "actions that are in character."[15] "Authenticity" generally connotes something authoritative, genuine, and true. In the present context, the patient's expressed preferences or behaviors are authentic only if the person is acting in character by making choices that are consistent with what would reasonably be expected based on past performance. Authenticity is more than mere *freedom* to choose; it is choice in the person that represents the person *faithfully*, by expressing settled preferences and beliefs, as contrasted with actions and choices motivated by desires and aversions of a momentary, brief, or fleeting duration.

Ambivalence by patients often presents the physician with questions about whether an apparent intention expresses the real will of the person. The patient, like all persons, is not simply a bundle of individual behaviors; every patient has a self or character developed through time. We can ask what the person would accept, want, or reject in a calm and deliberate moment when not under the sway of a momentary desire. Jackson and Youngner have argued that the "true autonomy" of patients consists in what they would want if they were in a calm, deliberate state.[16]

We must be careful, however, in bringing this conclusion to bear on actual medical practice. In effect, we argued in chapter four that it is easy for physicians to substitute (1) a determination of what the patient needs from the perspective of the beneficence model for (2) what the patient would prefer in a cool and informed moment. While it is true that the patient is not always the best judge of what is in his or her *best interests*, as determined by the beneficence model, the patient is the best judge of what he or she *wants* as determined by the autonomy model. It would be an insidious form of paternalism simply to substitute (1) for (2), and this substitution is far from what we are advocating in suggesting that stable values and preferences count for more than momentary ones or those that are unclear because of a patient's ambivalence or presentation of conflicting signals.

We do not even wish to argue that authenticity is a necessary condition of true autonomy. It is not. The important point about stable values is that if a person is acting out of character it would be irresponsible not to probe further for an explanation of the person's behavior, rather than simply ac-

[14]Ibid.

[15]See Gerald Dworkin, "Autonomy and Behavior Control," *Hastings Center Report* 6 (February 1976): 23–28; Bruce L. Miller, "Autonomy and the Refusal of Lifesaving Treatment," *Hastings Center Report* 11 (August 1981): 22–28; and James F. Childress, *Who Should Decide?: Paternalism and Health Care* (New York: Oxford University Press, 1982), pp. 63–65, 168.

[16]Jackson and Youngner, "Commentary: Family Wishes and Patient Autonomy," 22.

cepting an expression of immediate preference. Such behavior is a *warning* that a patient may not be acting autonomously, but until the person's reasons are known, we cannot simply override his or her preferences as if true autonomy had vanished. Once we ascertain the person's reasons, it may turn out that behavior and choices seemingly out of character are genuinely autonomous. The physican must also carefully avoid selecting which among a confusing pattern of conflicting intentions presented by the patient makes the most sense to the physician, because such a selection places him or her in the situation of acting solely as an agent of the beneficence model. This point is worth underscoring, because physicians typically worry about the patient's degree of autonomy when he or she refuses indicated care. Patients can also nonautonomously accept care.

To hold that the autonomy of patients should be understood in terms of a patient's stable and considered values is not to imply that these values must be a permanent feature of the patient's life. Such values may be open to change, even during the course of an illness. The salient criterion is that autonomous decisions must genuinely be the patient's own, and not simply the outcome of the oppression of disease or the constraining control of other persons. Reductions in autonomy are also not to be determined by values that the patient *ought* to have, based on such objective criteria as those constitutive of the beneficence model. Siegler has argued that some patients in "acute, critical, treatable" cases exhibit a strong capacity for autonomous choice, while others make "choices" on a quite irrational basis. He has no hesitation about "forcing" treatments on patients in the latter condition.[17] Of course, neither Siegler nor Jackson and Youngner hold that illness and its sequelae *necessarily* result in reductions of patient autonomy. Patients have different levels of resistance and control, and illness and its consequences do not by themselves provide unrestrained license for interventions. These physicians simply argue that the experience of physicians and patients alike teaches that autonomy can be reduced by illness and injury, and sometimes reduced substantially.[18]

Criteria of Reduced Autonomy

Our analysis in chapters one through four indicates that in order to qualify as autonomous, a person's decisions must (1) be based on adequate knowledge, (2) exhibit understanding and related intentionality, (3) not be internally constrained, and (4) not be externally constrained. A person's auton-

[17]On the latter point, see Mark Siegler and Ann Dudley Goldblatt, "Clinical Intuition: A Procedure for Balancing the Rights of Patients and the Responsibilities of Physicians," in *The Law-Medicine Relation: A Philosophical Exploration*, ed. S. F. Spicker, J. M. Healey, Jr., and H. Tristram Engelhardt, Jr. (Boston: D. Reidel Publishing Company, 1981), pp. 5–31.

[18]For a related account of the phenomenology of illness, see Edmund D. Pellegrino and David C. Thomasma, *A Philosophical Basis of Medical Practice: Toward a Philosophy and Ethic of the Healing Professions* (New York: Oxford University Press, 1981), esp. Chapter 9.

omy or self-governance is weakened and perhaps destroyed as these conditions go unsatisfied or are only weakly satisfied. The weaker an information base or a person's ability to understand and form intentions, for example, the weaker in autonomy is a decision made on this basis. Using this understanding of autonomy, we propose the following four criteria as the essential ingredients in any analysis of reduced autonomy.

1. Knowledge.   Can the patient grasp the relevant facts regarding his or her condition and diagnosis and treatment options? If not, the lack of information may constrain the person's choices. Here, the physician should not emphasize a particular ignorance or knowledge generally, but the psychological *ability* to marshal the knowledge required for the decision at hand. The crucial matter is not whether the patient does or does not presently have knowledge of relevant facts, but whether the patient could obtain such knowledge if the relevant information were available. If the patient lacks knowledge but could possess it, his or her autonomy is reduced by the lack of information, but the reduction can readily be eliminated by providing the relevant information. If the patient cannot—even with assistance—assimilate the information, his or her knowledge problem cannot (at that point in time) be overcome. On this criterion, Mrs. Simpson is reduced in her autonomy, perhaps substantially, while Mrs. Babcock and Mr. Perry appear to be autonomous.

2. Understanding.   Is the patient capable of cognitively appreciating received information and the consequences of his or her condition and diagnosis and treatment options? If not, the lack of understanding may constrain the person's choices. Here, one is assessing the patient's ability to understand and form intentions, as well as to project into the future and assess that future in terms of his or her values. If a patient's ability to understand is compromised, the connection between his or her values and decisions is threatened, and autonomy is reduced. Culver, Ferrell, and Green have argued that a patient allowed to decide about treatment should minimally understand (a) that the physician believes that treatment is needed and will aid the patient and (b) that he or she (the patient) is being asked to make a decision about a treatment.[19] While (a) and (b) are not jointly sufficient to assure substantial autonomy, the *absence* of this basic level of understanding is sufficient to indicate nonautonomy, not merely reduced autonomy. Developmental immaturity, psychiatric disorders, organic brain disease, and drugs all can affect understanding, as we are using the term. In the case of Mrs. Simpson, her inability to appreciate the consequences of failing to confirm a possible diagnosis of lung cancer renders her reduced in autonomy. This criterion of reduced autonomy does not appear to apply to Mrs. Babcock and Mr. Perry.

[19]Charles M. Culver, Richard B. Ferrell, and Ronald M. Green, "ECT and Special Problems of Informed Consent," *American Journal of Psychiatry* 137 (May 1980): 586–91.

3. Absence of Controlling Internal Constraints.   Is the patient controlled by internal forces that he or she is not capable of resisting? Such forces might constrain choice or cause a patient to make a decision that does not reflect his or her stable values or reasoned position. Such decisions are alien, not the patient's *own*. Internal constraints can also destabilize a patient's values. Changes brought on by serious acute illness or substantial medical interventions may be so profound as to overwhelm a patient's settled values, if the patient has any relevant and stable values. Key factors include sequelae of illness and medical interventions, such as pain, suffering, fear, and depression—precisely the sorts of factors identified by Jackson and Youngner. Applying this criterion is a complex matter: On the one hand, internal constraints might only temporarily constrain a patient's decision, as might be the case for Mr. Perry. On the other hand, these internal forces may be such that the patient cannot resist them. Depression and fear, of the sort that may be afflicting Mrs. Babcock, provide an example. Other examples are provided by patients locked into a psychological state of denial, as is characteristic, for example, of alcoholics.

4. Absence of Controlling External Constraints.   Is the patient's decision controlled by external forces or influences that the patient is not capable of resisting? Such forces might constrain choice or cause a patient to make a decision that does not reflect his or her values, perhaps because of irresistible dependence on the values of others. This may, for example, be the case with Mr. Perry, who seems deeply disturbed by his wife's ambivalence toward him. Key factors include the way the patient is affected by the impact of illness, treatment prognoses, hospitalization, and the like. Powerful authority figures, especially the physician, can function as controlling external constraints, as can coercive pressures, foreclosed options, compromising manipulations, behavior control techniques and the like.

These criteria indicate that reductions in autonomy come by degrees. The degree of reduction must be determined in specific contexts and in light of specific tasks. Fear of dying a painful and protracted death, as in the case of Mr. Perry, might reduce the autonomy of one patient, while leaving the autonomy of another substantially intact. An individual patient may lack understanding in some matters but not in others, and the lack may or may not be reversible.

Because reductions in autonomy come by degrees, a warning is appropriate regarding dangerous flexibility that can be built into the criteria we have proposed. One physician, Professor Milton Corn, has cautioned us that categories pertaining to "psychological pressures" can blemish a book in medical ethics like leprous sores, for they can function to permit the physician time and again to climb to safety over a straw bridge of speculation about psychological consequences of illness, hospitalization, and other forms of medical intervention. The physician is thus enabled to rationalize almost anything merely in order to avoid some anxiety or to produce some relief for a patient. Just as we cautioned in chapter four about the flexibility all too apparent in strong paternalism, so we must issue a warning here in the strongest terms about the use in medicine of judgments of future psychological states. The prediction of states of mind is not medical science—or any kind of science, for that matter—and psychiatry is often in no position to offer assistance. Medicine would do well to follow the law's firm principle that "a person is presumed to be competent unless shown *by evidence* not to be competent."[20]

This observation leads directly to problems of the patient's "competence" to decide and the evidence required for judgments of incompetence.

COMPETENCE AND INCOMPETENCE: THE LANGUAGE OF MEDICINE AND LAW

The language of reduced and substantially reduced autonomy has emerged largely from philosophical ethics and contemporary medical ethics. It has parallels, however, in the language of competence and incompetence in medicine and law. We turn now to determinations of competence and incompetence in these fields and to their bearing on determinations of reduced autonomy.

In its psychiatric and legal uses, the word "competence" is embedded in social practices whose history has spawned layers of meaning connected in diverse ways—layers formed because medicine, law, psychiatry, philosophy, and other professions and disciplines have had special interests in, and competing theories of, the abilities persons must have to be competent. But the *concept* of competence ranging across these different theories is nonetheless identical: *Competence is the ability to perform a task.*[21] These tasks need not be performed autonomously; indeed a performance could be nonautonomous but competent—as when a person skillfully performs some task while under hypnosis or while coerced by another person. One might also be incompetent to do something yet act autonomously in attempting it.

---

[20]See, e.g., *Lane v. Candura*, 376 N.E.2d 1232. This same position is defended in the context of moral theory by Childress, *Who Should Decide?: Paternalism in Health Care*, pp. 104f., 111, 169, 232f.

[21]Our analysis here and elsewhere in this section is indebted at several points to Bernard Gert and Charles Culver, "Competence to Consent: A Philosophical Overview," in *Competency and Informed Consent*, ed. Natalie Reatig (Rockville, MD.: National Institute of Mental Health, 1981), pp. 12–31; and as subsequently revised and expanded in their *Philosophy in Medicine: Conceptual and Ethical Issues in Medicine and Psychiatry* (New York: Oxford University Press, 1982), Chapter 3. Culver and Gert argue in the latter work (pp. 53–54) that competence "is not merely a synonym for ability" and that "two necessary features for being competent to perform an activity are that one understands what that activity is and knows when he is performing it."

We often censure the autonomous behavior of others by using the label "incompetent." Whereas autonomy is self-governance and reduced autonomy is reduced self-governance, competence is the ability to perform a task and diminished competence is a diminished or lesser ability to perform it. Clearly, then, autonomy and competence are distinct concepts. Yet they are commonly conflated in law, medicine, and medical ethics, as if they were the same concept. The reason for this conflation, we believe, is the following: If one's self-governance (autonomy) is reduced, it is highly likely (although not necessary) that one's ability to perform certain tasks also will be diminished. Thus, a reduction of autonomy can easily cause diminished competence, especially in decisionmaking. We shall be in a better position to understand this connection between reduced autonomy and diminished competence after further exploration of the nature of the concept of competence.

The Concept of Competence

All judgments of competence require the specification of a context, of relevant abilities, of the stability of the abilities at a time, and of some threshold degree of possession of the abilities. We shall consider these four dimensions of the concept individually.

1. The Context. A judgment of competence is senseless unless made particular in a context. If a physician says about the first case, "Mrs. Simpson is incompetent," the most natural response is, "Mrs. Simpson is incompetent to do what?" The *what* must then be specified: to manage her legal affairs? to recognize her daughter? to remember her medical history? or to decide about bronchoscopy? Depending on the particular context, Mrs. Simpson could be competent or incompetent. The *concept* of competence, however, is indifferent to which particular context is specified.

While it is meaningful to describe persons as *generally* competent, this judgment, too, assumes a context: the ordinary affairs of life. Only rarely do we judge someone competent or incompetent as regards (virtually) every ordinary sphere of life. Such a judgment is usually irrelevant in medicine, for the physician is likely to be investigating some particular competence, such as competence to decide about a particular diagnostic measure or a particular treatment regimen. All three of our cases feature this question about competence. If we ask whether such patients are able to make informed choices, we do not usually mean "able to make informed choices generally." Certainly this is not in doubt in Mr. Perry's case. Rather we mean "informed choices of a certain kind"—e.g., about a drug regimen, as in the case of Mrs. Babcock, or to be "no coded" in Mr. Perry's case. These cases show how the concept of competence is inherently context-specific.

2. Relevant Abilities. The abilities generally looked for in judgments of competence—especially in medical settings— are abilities of a psychological character. If Mr. Perry, an accountant, is competent to prepare tax returns, then he has the psychological abilities required to do so. If Mrs. Babcock is competent to fight off depression, then she has the psychological reserves necessary to do so—whatever those abilities are. Therefore, to establish whether someone is competent or incompetent to perform some specific task, the psychological abilities required by that task in the context must be established, and one must also establish whether the person possesses these abilities. Hence, the concept of competence is ability-specific.

3. Stability and Variability of the Abilities. Even when judgments of competence are afforded a well-defined context and a particular set of psychological abilities to perform a specific task, competence is not fixed across time. The same person can at the same time be incompetent to perform some tasks and competent to perform others, and a person can be incompetent to do something at one point in time and perfectly competent to perform that same task at another point in time. For example, in a precedent legal case on the capacity of mental patients to consent, a court was perplexed by a highly intelligent patient who was at times competent to refuse medication and at other times not, "depending on the day."[22] A single individual's ability to consent, refuse, resist, or decide may vary over time—which is why the designation "intermittent" is appropriate in Mrs. Simpson's case. Thus, she might at one particular time be competent to decide whether to accept various interventions, while at other times she might be questionably competent to do so. This is precisely the situation confronting Mrs. Simpson's physician. Hence, like the concept of autonomy, the concept of competence involves questions of stability and permanence.

These second and third points may seem trivial, but, as Jeffrie Murphy has pointed out,[23] statutory laws commonly assume that a person who is incompetent to make medical decisions or to conduct various affairs that create self-danger is equally incompetent to vote, manage bank accounts, get married, and the like. But the assertion "Person X is incompetent to do some particular Y and therefore not responsible for doing Y" should never carry the automatic implication that X is not competent for *any other* decision or action. Such judgments are patently unreasonable and fly in the face of what we know about the etiology of various forms of incompetence. Physicians who work with patients in extreme pain, such as Mr. Perry, can well appreciate the intermittent character that competence sometimes assumes. We all appreciate how children and adults in learning situations develop competencies over time. For example, children in early stages of cognitive development are incompetent to perform various cognitive tasks that they later master easily. These considerations suggest—indeed compel—

---

[22]*Rennie v. Klein* 462 F. Supp. 1131 (1978).

[23]Jeffrie G. Murphy, "Incompetence and Paternalism," in his *Retribution, Justice, and Therapy: Essays in the Philosophy of Law* (Boston: D. Reidel Publishing Co., 1979), pp. 166–67.

precise statements about the decisions persons are expected to be able to make.

4. Degree of Possession of the Abilities.   Competence is also a continuum concept: A judgment of more or less competence can be made, as can a judgment of diminished or increased competence. Like autonomy, competence is not an either/or phenomenon. There is a meaningful sense in which we can say not only that someone is competent to do something, but also that the person is more competent or less competent to do it than someone else—or even more or less competent than the person himself or herself used to be, for competence with respect to a task may fluctuate significantly over time. Such judgments are possible because the required abilities can be possessed to a greater or lesser extent. For example, a pulmonary specialist may be more competent to consent to bronchoscopy for himself than is Mrs. Simpson; but Mrs. Simpson may be more competent than the specialist to help prepare a meal for a family of five, even with all her medical problems. In any given treatment context it should be ascertained precisely which decisions or actions are in question, while avoiding the simplistic dichotomy of "either competent or incompetent."

In various practical contexts, we must create cutoffs on the continuum from full competence through partial competence to complete incompetence. Such cutoffs allow us to say that any person past a certain point should be treated as incompetent. Mr. Perry seems not to be incompetent in this sense, but Mrs. Simpson may be. In making these broad judgments, we transform competence from a *continuum* concept to a *threshold* concept. Everyone on the "competence side" is classified as equally competent.[24] However, not only is it patently false in most contexts that individuals are equally competent, it is often a fragile matter how and where the threshold marking incompetence is to be established, and borderline cases are virtually always unavoidable.

We conclude that the concept of competence is defined by the four central characteristics delineated in this section and that these characteristics conform to the use of "competence" in professional contexts and ordinary-language contexts alike. In both, the core meaning of "competence" is the ability to perform a specific task. This analysis of competence also suffices for incompetence: A person is incompetent if not competent, and compe-

---

[24]This distinction is explored in Daniel Wikler, "Paternalism and the Mildly Retarded," *Philosophy and Public Affairs* 8 (Summer 1979): 377–92, and reissued as "The Bright Man's Burden," in *Mental Retardation and Sterilization: A Problem of Competency and Paternalism*, ed. R. Macklin and W. Gaylin (New York: Plenum Press, 1981), Chapter 10, pp. 149–66. Wikler distinguishes a *relativist* conception of competence (people are *more or less* competent) from a *threshold* conception (people above the threshold are *equally* competent). These two conceptions are mutually exclusive as Wikler analyzes them. However, if the "*equally* competent" provision is dropped in favor of "*sufficiently* competent," the two conceptions are consistent. Our analysis uses precisely this strategy.

tent if not incompetent. Someone is incompetent if he or she cannot perform a task at the required threshold level on a performance continuum. An individual may only temporarily suffer impairment of needed cognitive or affective abilities or may suffer permanent, irreversible impairment. In principle, once a threshold has been fixed, it should be possible to establish by empirical investigation whether a person is psychologically incompetent in either of these two respects.

This analysis also reveals important dissimilarities between the concepts of diminished competence and reduced autonomy. The conditions of nonconstraint (internal and external) found in analyses of autonomy are seldom invoked in discussions of competence because a person can sometimes perform competently even if constrained. Also, legal criteria of rational decisionmaking that have proven influential in judgments of competence have played no *parallel* role in analyses of autonomy. These criteria play a pervasive role in clinical judgment, and thus deserve further consideration.

Criteria of Incompetence

Inappropriate Criteria. We can easily be misled in the quest for the range of abilities required for patients to make competent decisions about diagnosis and treatment. We often speak, for example, of a person as incompetent to decide about something if he or she lacks critical information. Someone might say that Mr. Perry is incompetent because he lacks information about what the future holds for him or lacks information about the counseling his wife might receive. Building on this usage, Jeffrie Murphy has made *ignorance* one of three primary conditions of incompetence to make decisions. He argues that a patient is incompetent to make a decision about brain surgery, for example, "because he lacks the kind of knowledge that is relevant to making a decision of this sort."[25] Murphy is using the notion of a lack or insufficiency of *knowledge* as the basis of a theory of incompetence, whereas we have used lack of psychological *ability* as basic. Murphy's proposal seems to express the "informed" part of the informed decisionmaking process we discussed in chapter three, where we also noticed that a lack of information can lead to questions about the inability of patients to assume responsibility for a decision. Do we, then, need Murphy's analysis of informational deficiency in addition to our analysis in terms of task-specific abilities?

As a matter of the broad use of "incompetence" in the English language, Murphy is correct: It is logically possible that persons might be incompetent owing to ignorance, for ignorance can render a person *unable* to decide. Moreover, as Alan Meisel and Loren Roth correctly note, there is a

---

[25]Murphy, "Incompetence and Paternalism," p. 167.

strong "conceptual overlap" between "competency and understanding."[26] We believe, however, that a person's competence to decide is not contingent upon the present state of a person's information. It is centrally a matter of his or her psychological abilities to possess the information, whether it is possessed or not. Competence turns on the ability or capacity to process information, and in this sense to understand. We can consistently say that someone is competent to (able to) decide even though presently ignorant (and for that reason unable). We mean that the person does not lack the psychological abilities necessary for deciding. Instead, he or she lacks—and requires—information. If there is ignorance based on the inability to process information, then this inability *would* constitute incompetence.

Just as ignorance is not to be confused with incompetence in our analysis, so we must not confuse other factors with conditions that render a person incompetent. For example, in a widely cited legal decision, a Michigan court held that a mentally disturbed prisoner did not have the ability to make a treatment decision because "the very nature of his incarceration diminished the capacity to consent to psychosurgery. He is particularly vulnerable as a result of his mental condition, the deprivation stemming from involuntary confinement, and the effects of the phenomenon of institutionalization."[27] This statement has been criticized for confusing freedom of choice with the question of mental capacity and for implying that a potentially coercive environment can render an otherwise competent person *incompetent* to make decisions regarding his or her best interests.[28] We do not share these criticisms because we understand the court to assert only that all three of the distinct conditions it cites jointly render the person *vulnerable*—a view that we find congenial. The important matter is that even a highly coercive environment does not necessarily render a person's particular decision *incompetent*—not even if the environment coerces other choices.

Appropriate Criteria.   Having now outlined the criteria that are not appropriate to the concepts of competence and incompetence, we must outline appropriate criteria. These criteria center on the various abilities

---

[26]Alan Meisel and Loren H. Roth, "What We Do and Do Not Know about Informed Consent," *Journal of the American Medical Association* 246 (27 November 1981): 2473–77 at 2474; and "Tests of Competency to Consent to Treatment" (with Charles W. Lidz), *American Journal of Psychiatry* 134 (March 1977): 279–84. See also Meisel's "Legal Overview," in *Competency and Informed Consent*, ed. N. Reatig, pp. 32–71.

[27]*Kaimowitz v. Department of Mental Health*, Civil No. 73-19434-AW (Circuit Court, Wayne County, Mich., July 10, 1973), pp. 31–32. Summarized at 42 U.S.L.W. 3064 (July 31, 1973) and reprinted in U.S. Senate, Committee on the Judiciary, Subcommittee on Constitutional Rights, *Individual Rights and the Federal Role in Behavior Modification* (Washington: U.S. Government Printing Office, 1974), pp. 510–24. But see *Rogers v. Okin* (note 34), for a contrasting view.

[28]See Paul S. Appelbaum and Loren H. Roth, "Competency to Consent to Research: A Psychiatric Overview," *Archives of Genral Psychiatry* 39 (August 1982): 951–58; also in *Competency and Informed Consent*, ed. N. Reatig, pp. 72–105; and Jeffrie G. Murphy, "Therapy and the Problem of Autonomous Consent," *International Journal of Law and Psychiatry* 2 (1979): 415–30.

required for decisionmaking. A wide variety of criteria specifying how incompetence to decide is to be determined has been suggested in literature on the subject, e.g., in discussion of mental status examinations.[29] However, in some surveys of the literature on competence and informed consent, Roth, Meisel, and their colleagues at the University of Pittsburgh have discovered seven pervasively operative categories of "tests" of incompetence.[30] These important tests merit individual review. (We have slightly reorganized and reconstructed their analysis.)

1. *Absence of Decision.* This first test is simple: Can the person evidence a choice? This criterion focuses not on the quality of a decision but rather on the sheer absence or presence of a decision by the patient—e.g., a preference for treatment—as well as the communication of a decision. If the patient cannot evidence a choice—say yes or no, shake his or her head, or engage in some other meaningful behavioral equivalent—the patient is incompetent. The person's understanding or informed decisionmaking is not tested.

2. *General Inability to Understand.* This criterion tests whether the patient has the *ability,* rather than the actual understanding, to understand the nature of his or her situation. The determination of this ability is usually made inferentially through intelligence tests, mental status examinations, and the like. The ability to understand and assess risks, benefits, and alternatives to treatment is emphasized in decisionmaking contexts in medicine. Precise or perfect understanding is not required; only fundamental cognitive abilities must be possessed.

3. *Inability to Understand Disclosed Information.* The third criterion tests whether the patient is able to understand the meaning of the information provided in the professional's disclosure. Often this is determined by whether the patient did in fact understand, rather than whether the person is generally able to understand. Neither here nor in the previous test is the person's weighing of the information to be evaluated. Mrs. Simpson might be incompetent under this criterion.

4. *Failure to Articulate a Reason.* Failure to articulate a reason in support of the decision refers to the patient able to evidence a choice but unable to give any reason for the choice.

5. *Failure to Give a Rational Reason.* In the fifth test, the patient is able to give a reason, but not a rational one. An obvious problem is how one defines "rational," and sharp argument surrounds whether an act such as Mr. Perry's suicide would be based on a rational reason. Usually a minimal notion of rationality is used. For example, there must be some plausible connection between the reason and the choice. Quality of thought is presumably the determinant, although no one has been able to delineate satisfactorily the

[29]See Thomas P. Detre and David J. Kupfer, "Psychiatric History and The Mental Status Examination," in *Comprehensive Textbook of Psychiatry,* 2nd ed., ed. A. M. Freedman, H. I. Kaplan, and B. J. Sadock (Baltimore: Williams & Wilkins, 1975), pp. 724–33.

[30]Roth and Meisel, "What We Do and Do Not Know about Informed Consent." See also Appelbaum and Roth, "Competency to Consent to Research: A Psychiatric Overview," passim, and the earlier article by Roth, Meisel, and Lidz, "Tests of Competency to Consent to Treatment," 279–84. For a thoughtful approach to a similar range of tests that relates to our discussion of informed consent in chapter three, see Ruth Macklin, "Some Problems in Gaining Informed Consent from Psychiatric Patients," *Emory Law Journal* 31 (Spring 1982): 360–68.

difference between a rational and a nonrational reason, and disagreements abound over problems of subjective assessments of rationality, the nature of mental illness, and the like.

6. *Failure to Employ a Risk/Benefit Calculus.* This test indicates that the patient failed to base the decision on a reasonable weighing of potential risks and potential benefits. Here the patient could have some rational reasons yet fail to employ risk/benefit comparisons. Thus this test is stiffer than those above. Quite possibly both Mrs. Simpson and Mrs. Babcock would be judged incompetent to decide their treatment by this test. This test also runs the risk of being the most arbitrary, because it requires a weighing of items already labeled risks and benefits—whether the patient sees them as risks and benefits or not.

7. *Nature of the Decision.* This test bases judgments of incompetence on the outcome chosen (consent or refusal), rather than on the process by which the decision was reached. Usually the appeal is to some external criterion—e.g., if the patient failed to choose what a reasonable person would choose in similar circumstances, the person is incompetent. The outcome might also be invalidated if no reasonable practitioner would sanction the choice as medically sound. This test is the one most likely to clash with the patient's autonomy. Mrs. Simpson, Mrs. Babcock, and Mr. Perry could all be found incompetent by some standard versions of this test.

It is useful to arrange these tests through the following table of generic and specific criteria of incompetence—all seven of which are currently in competition as *favored* reasons for considering a person incompetent to consent or refuse medical interventions and therapies:

A. ABSENCE OF A DECISION
1. The person is unable to evidence a choice.

B. ABSENCE OF AN ADEQUATE REASON (IN MAKING A DECISION)
2. The person is unable to give a supporting reason.
3. The person gives a reason but is unable to give a rational reason.
4. The person gives a rational reason but is unable to make risk/benefit judgments.

C. ABSENCE OF AN ADEQUATE UNDERSTANDING (IN MAKING A DECISION)
5. The person is unable to understand the situation.
6. The person is unable to understand disclosed information.

D. ABSENCE OF AN ADEQUATE OUTCOME (IN MAKING A DECISION)
7. The person is unable to reach a reasonable decision (as judged, e.g., by a reasonable person standard).

INTERVENTIONS BY PHYSICIANS

Problems in the Justification of Intervention

Our treatment of the concepts of autonomy and competence sets the stage for addressing the second question we posed at the beginning of this chapter: How should the physician treat a patient of reduced autonomy who has a relatively low degree of competence to decide about diagnosis and treatment? Consider again our three cases: Mrs. Simpson appears incompetent to decide about diagnostic bronchoscopy, or at least her daughter seems far more competent to make such a decision. What, then, is the morally responsible course for her physician to follow: How *may* the physician treat her, and how *should* the physician treat her? Moreover, are the standards for competence *to refuse* identical with standards for competence *to consent*? That is, should we say that a person is equally competent to consent or to refuse, and that we should honor (or not honor) the person's decision whether he or she refuses or consents?[31]

In the case of Mrs. Babcock, it is uncertain to what degree she might be competent to consent to the use of antidepressant drug therapy. Her requisite psychological capabilities might be diminished—either by environmental or organic factors. What, then, does morality demand or permit of her physician? Finally, in the case of Mr. Perry, we have an apparently competent choice for suicide and a request for noninterference. Does Mr. Perry's apparent competence alter the obligations suggested by the beneficence model? Does his competence render the autonomy model overriding? These questions cannot be answered by a simple appeal to criteria of incompetent decisions. Appeal to such guides is but the first step in the justification of an intervention.

In order to specify how "competence" judgments ought to function in medicine—e.g., by placing a label of "incompetence" on a patient—we must understand the potential train of paternalistic, coercive, and authorizing events that can be set in motion by using such labels. This is crucially the case when dealing with patients whose autonomy is reduced to an uncertain degree. As Jeffrie Murphy has argued, "The real problem that will face us, then, is what to do in the borderline cases. When in doubt, which way should we err—on the side of safety [as required by the beneficence model] or on the side of liberty [as required by the autonomy model]? It is vital that we do not adopt analyses of incompetence or patterns of argument that obscure the obviously moral nature of this question."[32] Incompetence judgments can presuppose moral judgments about whether to treat, just as easily as moral determinations about whether to treat can presuppose incompetence judgments. There is a constant interplay between them, and seldom will *empirical* determinations of the presence or absence of abilities be entirely nonevaluative.

A commitment to one or more of the tests of competence previously discussed inevitably carries some form of value commitment regarding

---

[31]Meisel and Roth have long defended the position that there should be symmetry in standards of competency for consent and competency for refusal. This position contrasts with reports from the President's Commission for the Study of Ethical Problems in Medicine and Biomedical and Behavioral Research, which takes the position that whether one is competent depends in part on what one decides.

[32]Murphy, "Incompetence and Paternalism," p. 174.

justified intervention. Those who accept a stringent test of incompetence (see #6 and #7, p. 124) favor an emphasis on the beneficence model by placing the medical interests and safety of patients above their liberty. A psychiatrist wedded to strong paternalism, for example is likely to adopt one of the stringent tests. By contrast, those committed more broadly to liberty and autonomy rights will judge that these values have priority over values of health and saftey—that is, that the autonomy model has priority over the beneficence model. This commitment will likely eventuate in the adoption of one of the less stringent tests of incompetence (see #1 through 5, p. 123–124). Conflicts based on these different commitments should come as no surprise, for they are simply one further example of the clash between the autonomy model and the beneficence model that we have repeatedly witnessed. While we cannot hope to completely eliminate disagreements as to which values should take priority, we can insist that the person who acts on either model, or some combination of the two, has carefully reasoned through the implications of his or her actions.

One might therefore be tempted to adopt the following general rule: *Justified* declarations of seriously diminished competence or incompetence provide sufficient justification for interventions on the patient's behalf. Although such a rule has implicitly been operative in medicine, it does *not* follow from the incompetence of a patient's decision that the decision may be justifiably overridden. The proper moral approach, instead, is one that balances the interests at stake in both the beneficence and autonomy models: If a patient is diminished in competence (in any of the several senses identified above) because capability for autonomous decisions is significantly reduced, the patient may be justifiably protected from harm that might result because of a compromised state. This compromised state does not, however justify the person's subjection to whatever form of medical benefit another might think good for the person. From the fact that Mrs. Simpson might be incompetent, it does not follow that her daughter or her physician should not abide by her wishes. In the case of many persons whom we justifiably hold to be incompetent, morality may require that we not intervene in their affairs. We should therefore be cautious not to assume any logical connection between incompetence and involuntary treatment or intervention.[33]

This point has been delicately handled in some recent court decisions. In *Rogers v. Okin*[34] a Massachusetts court ruled—to the consternation of many psychiatrists[35]—that hospitalized mental patients have a constitutional right to refuse coerced treatment, except under emergency conditions.

---

[33]See Ibid., 173, for a useful analysis.

[34]*Rogers v. Okin*, 634 F.2d 650 (1980) and 478 F. Supp. 1342 (1979). U.S. cert granted April 20, 1981. But see the *Kaimowitz* case noted above.

[35]See P. Schaffer, *Clinical Psychiatry News* 8 (January 1980): 1.

The case turned on the forced injection of psychotropic medication[36] to which a patient vigorously objected. Defendant psychiatrists and hospital officials in the case maintained that "a committed mental patient is *per se* incompetent to decide whether or not to receive treatment" and that the professional's duty is to provide the best possible treatment irrespective of the patient's expressed desires, even if patients have the ability to act freely.[37] The American Psychiatric Association filed a statement in the case arguing that "the decision to *commit* a person against his will . . . [seems] a sufficient constitutional predicate to justify the provision of that *treatment* for which the individual was committed to receive."[38] However, responses based on this premise may be an indiscriminate conflation of different abilities to choose and thus blind us to the fact that while these patients may be unable to choose, act, and assume responsibility in many contexts of life, they may well be capable of some important autonomous decisions. Such decisions may help preserve what little dignity remains to them in stark institutional settings.

The United States Supreme Court ultimately remanded *Rogers v. Okin,*[39] and a more important case turned out to be *Guardianship of Roe,* which also originated in Massachusetts and which relied extensively on certain findings in *Rogers.* The court in this case addressed the question of whether the father and guardian of a person who is mentally ill and unable to care for himself possesses the authority to consent to the forcible administration of antipsychotic medication. The son and ward was not institutionalized and not in emergency circumstances. The son had been convicted of several criminal offenses and refused strongly recommended medication (Haldol and Prolixin). The court argued that "absent an overwhelming State interest, a competent individual has the right to refuse such treatment." To

---

[36]Psychotropic medications are drugs that affect the psyche. These particular drugs were "antipsychotic," which for the court referred to Thorazine, Mellaril, Prolixin, and Haldol.

[37]*Rogers v. Okin,* pp. 1360–67. The psychiatrists also contended in this case that it would be an administrative nightmare to permit refusals of treatment by committed patients—no doubt a significant practical problem.

[38]*Rogers v. Okin,* fn. 4. U.S. Court of Appeals (First Circuit) rejected this reasoning on grounds that a finding of mental illness is not "equivalent to a finding that the individual is incapable of deciding for himself whether commitment and treatment are in his own best interest." The court notes that there is a "profound distinction" between commitment and determination of competency. The Canadian Psychiatric Association was at the same time defending the opposite point of view. See C. H. Cahn, "Consent in Psychiatry: The Position of the Canadian Psychiatric Association," *Canadian Journal of Psychiatry* 25 (February 1980): 78–85, esp. 83.

[39]*Mills v. Rogers,* 101 S.Ct. 2442 (1982), 682 Ed. 2d 293 (1981). On June 18, 1982 the Supreme Court *vacated* the Court of Appeals decisions in *Rogers v. Okin* and remanded the case to see whether intervening in Massachusetts *state* law (exemplified by then in *Guardianship of Roe* cited in note 40) might affect the case. The opinions in *Rogers v. Okin* now have no legal or precedental effect. The Supreme Court also held that Massachusetts may have recognized broader liberty interests *of the incompetent* than the liberty interests protected by the U.S. Constitution.

deny persons this right is to "degrade" them, making them wholly reliant on other persons. The court goes out of its way to "emphasize that the determination being made is *not* what is medically in the ward's best interests."[40]

This court held that five factors must be weighed against the expressed preferences of the patient and ward: (1) the intrusiveness of the proposed treatment, (2) the possibility of adverse side effects, (3) the absence of an emergency, (4) prior judicial involvement, and (5) the likelihood of conflicting interests. The court held that "even if the ward lacks capacity to make treatment decisions, his stated preference is entitled to serious consideration as a factor in the substituted judgment determination" by a guardian; indeed, the court says these preferences should shape our very understanding of "his 'best interests'." Religious and other beliefs are to be accepted with equal seriousness. The court holds that while the state could on some occasion have compelling reasons for requiring the medication (e.g., to prevent violence), the basic standard of justification for forced medication is the same as the standard for denying liberty in cases of involuntary commitment. The court therefore allowed the father to continue to be the guardian, but refused to authorize involuntary treatment.[41] Such judicial findings have been severely criticized in some psychiatric and medical circles.[42]

Guides for Intervention

Judgments of diminished competence, then, do not automatically justify interventions directed by the beneficence model. Intervention with patients whose *autonomy* is reduced must be guided by *both* models. The two models together suggest three guides for intervention with patients afflicted by reduced autonomy.[43]

---

[40]*In the Matter of Guardianship of Richard Roe III.* Mass. 421 N.E.2d 40 (Supreme Judicial Court of Massachusetts, 1981), pp. 51–52. This case was decided *before* the Supreme Court vacated the court of appeals decision in *Rogers v. Okin.*

[41]*Guardianship of Roe,* pp. 57–62.

[42]See an early and influential criticism by Harvey Shwed, "Social Policy and the Rights of the Mentally Ill: Time for Re-examination," *Journal of Health Politics, Policy, and Law* 5 (1980): 193ff. Predictably he questions whether an autonomous decision can be made by many psychiatric patients even if they are legally competent.

[43]The guides that we propose seem to contrast with others, notably those of the President's Commission for the Study of Ethical Problems in Medicine and Biomedical and Behavioral Research, *Making Health Care Decisions,* pp. 177–88. However, their standards are for "surrogate decisionmaking," whereas ours are guides for intervention by physicians. We are not suggesting that a physician should be the proxy decisionmaker or even that a justified intervention by physicians should override the competing decision of a legally authorized decisionmaker. See also the Commission's *Deciding to Forego Life-Sustaining Treatment* (Washington, D.C.: U.S. Government Printing Office, 1983), p. 5. The Commission recommends that an appropriate surrogate be named to make decisions regarding treatment. Two guides are proposed. First, the surrogate should attempt to "replicate the [decisions] the pa-

Guide 1. The first guide applies to patients with reversibly reduced autonomy: The strained or broken connection between their values and decisions can be restored. This guide is based on the autonomy model and directs the physician to restore the patient's capability for autonomous decisions. As the patient improves, his or her choices are to be given increasing weight, as demanded by an increased level of autonomy. Consider Mr. Perry's request not to be resuscitated if he attempts suicide. A single-minded use of the autonomy model would assert that patients have a right to end their lives, provided no significant harm befalls others. Because Mr. Perry's family presumably will not know that his death is the result of suicide and because further psychological and financial harm to them would be prevented, the physician's moral responsibility is not to interfere with Mr. Perry. This conclusion is sustainable, however, only on the assumption that Mr. Perry's pain, his concern about his financial condition, and his deeply strained relationship with his wife have no constraining impact on his decisionmaking abilities. The more we ascertain autonomy to be reduced, the greater is the physician's obligation to intervene in order to assess Mr. Perry's ability to make autonomous decisions. One would do so not because Mr. Perry wants to commit suicide, but rather because there is evidence that some of the four criteria for reduced autonomy might apply in his case.

If Mr. Perry's decision turns out to be autonomous, then rejecting it simply because its underlying values conflict with the values of the beneficence model would constitute an invalid invocation of strong paternalism. The concerns of autonomy are not minimal in this case: Mr. Perry's choices are of overwhelming significance because they are based on his values and beliefs about the quality of his remaining life, the tenor of his relationship with his wife, and the future well-being of his family. Mr. Perry's choice to commit suicide is surely an unusual choice; it deeply offends the life-preserving directives of the beneficence model. Yet the most that can be concluded about his decision is that it is drastic in its consequence, and therefore forces serious examination of its basis.

While Mr. Perry is asking his physician to accept an obligation not to interfere with an act contrary to the most basic values of the beneficence model, the physican is no slave to this model. Two courses of action are consistent with the demands of both models. First, the physician might try to persuade Mr. Perry—through means short of a controlling external influence—to change his mind and discontinue treatment, rather than to commit suicide. The suggestion for delay by Jackson and Youngner would

---

tient would make if capable of doing so." The second guide applies when there is insufficient evidence about the patient's wishes. It directs the surrogate to act in the patient's best interests as these are understood from an objective viewpoint. These two guides parallel our second and third guides.

be pertinent and acceptable. Second, in the face of a firm decision by Mr. Perry for suicide, the physician should enter the no code order in Mr. Perry's chart, as requested. To do otherwise emphasizes too much the values of medicine over those of the patient, falling again into an unjustified strong paternalism. Of course, the physician would not be required to assist in Mr. Perry's suicide if he or she found it to be morally objectionable, e.g., on religious grounds. In these circumstances, it would be appropriate to refer Mr. Perry to a physician who has moral convictions that would not be violated by entering the no code order in Mr. Perry's chart.

Patients with reduced autonomy occasionally have provided their physicians with prior directives that some forms of treatment should not be administered. Such directives are expressions of the right to refuse medical interventions. Treatment that involved the prohibited interventions would be inconsistent with respect for the patient's autonomy, even if that treatment were intended to restore autonomy.

Guide 2.   In a second range of cases a different guide is called for: Autonomy cannot be restored, but a relevant and sufficiently complete set of the patient's values and beliefs can be constructed from prior autonomous determinations. To insist on respect for a patient's *autonomy* (in contrast to respect for *persons*) is an empty gesture in such cases, and it would at first seem that the physician must rely exclusively on the beneficence model. The problem with this justification is that the patient, were he or she autonomous, might balance the available goods and harms differently from the physician and might even reject the entire framework of the beneficence model.

Prior to his or her present condition of substantially reduced autonomy, the patient may have made autonomous choices relevant to the issue at hand. If ascertainable, such prior expression of the patient's autonomy should be respected. A patient's "value history"[44]—the analogue of the person's physical, mental, and sexual history—might be developed on the basis of what the physician knows about the patient and information obtained from family members (and perhaps from others who know the patient well). A decision regarding diagnosis or treatment could then be made consistent with this value history. No doubt this suggestion has severe and often insurmountable practical limits, for value histories are seldom specific or directly pertinent to such decisions. A platitude such as "he had a

---

[44]We borrow this phrase from Edmund Pellegrino. Robert Veatch discusses a similar notion of "the moral history of the individual" in his *A Theory of Medical Ethics,* p. 209. Veatch joins this notion with that of "moral communities for the individual." Developing the patient's value history would begin with a determination of the patient's values and beliefs about the goods and harms constitutive of the beneficence model and how they are to be weighted. It would then go on to identify other relevant values and beliefs. Family members would be a key source for the physician in this process. They would not be asked to decide about the patient's treatment, however. The basis for such decisions remains with the patient's prior autonomy.

zest for living" will not suffice as a basis for refusing a respirator. (Living wills have often been criticized for this reason, but they are sometimes considerably more specific as expressions of intention than are value histories.)

Consider the case of Mrs. Babcock, perhaps the most difficult of our three cases to analyze. Mrs. Babcock is distracted by her fear of death and abandonment. An organic condition, resulting in depression, could also be present. Is she thereby rendered nonautonomous? This question confronts her physician, and there is no ready, irrefutable answer. She occupies that "gray area" between some level of reduced autonomy and substantial autonomy. Suppose that Mrs. Babcock's decision can never be rendered substantially autonomous. In this event, the second guide indicates that the drug should probably be administered. Her value history shows some evidence of a previous willingness to accept such treatment. The drug could also be administered as a trial; if it fails to work, the problem can be reconsidered in light of the new information gathered in the meantime. Such decisions, once made, need not be made forever. Here, as elsewhere, the physician should be prepared to make adjustments in light of the patient's progress (or lack of it).

Guide 3. In the remaining cases, autonomy cannot be restored, and a value history cannot be obtained or reasonably reconstructed, or the patient may never have been autonomous, as in the case of the profoundly or severely retarded individual or a newborn infant. The autonomy model provides no guide in such cases, but the beneficence model provides guidance because it gives an objective account of the goods and harms that define *any* patient's best interests. The famous case of Joseph Saikewicz overtly calls for this third standard.[45] Given the severity of his mental retardation, it was impossible for Mr. Saikewicz to make an autonomous decision about the treatment of his leukemia, and no relevant value history could be provided. In such cases, physicians should look exclusively to the beneficence model. Contrary to the conclusion of the court in this case, the beneficence model might justify administration of chemotherapy because it holds out a thirty to fifty percent chance of remission of his disease.

CONCLUSION

In this chapter we have considered how the moral demands of beneficence and respect for autonomy apply in circumstances of reduced autonomy and diminished competence. We have argued that as the patient's auton-

---

[45]*Superintendent of Belchertown v. Saikewicz*, Mass. 370 N.E.2d 417 (1977). See note 21 in chapter 4 of this text. The court does not agree with our exclusion of the autonomy model because it relies heavily on the legal principle of substituted judgment, an autonomy-based standard.

omy is reduced and the need for care increases, the moral demand to respect autonomy progressively recedes in significance; but to the extent the patient's autonomy is intact, the justification for intervention in the name of beneficence becomes progressively more difficult. This conclusion develops naturally from the argument in chapter four. We have argued in both chapters that various unauthorized interventions by physicians can be justified, and may be laudatory, including some that qualify as strong paternalism.[46] We have at the same time cautioned against overinterpretation of the moral warrants that support the physician in intervening against the expressed preferences of patients—e.g., by presuming that the physician has a *right* to intervene.

The other side of this warning, which we have not emphasized in either of these chapters, but might have, is the problem of individual judgment and uncertainty that confronts the physician in clinical practice. Decisionmaking for incapacitated patients is an extremely complex problem for which law, medicine, and philosophy have yet to find entirely adequate answers. It is important to bear this in mind when criticizing the actions of others. Moreover, if a patient presents with acute onset of a serious illness, the physician has no opportunity for a relaxed philosophical inquiry into the state of the patient's autonomy. The patient with a serious, acute illness, suffering from fear and pain, requires immediate attention, sometimes by overriding the patient's frustrated objections. Physicians in such circumstances are surely to be forgiven if they occasionally overinterpret the dictates of the beneficence model, for it is we who have given them this awesome responsibility. The physician is charged to preserve life and health as well as to respect autonomy, and it must not be forgotten how very difficult this dual obligation can be in circumstances of uncertain medical evidence and ambivalence in a patient with reduced autonomy.

[46]We have not argued in either chapter that such interventions are morally *obligatory* because of the professional role of the physician—a more difficult thesis to prove, and one that we shall have to postpone for some future occasion. Some reflections on this problem—with conclusions different from the one we would reach—are found in Childress, *Who Should Decide?: Paternalism in Health Care*, p. 116f.

Chapter 6

Third-Party
Interests

In previous chapters we examined the physician's responsibilities largely under the assumption of a one-to-one relationship: a particular physician responding to a particular patient. We have examined to some extent the family's role in patient care, but we have not directly considered third parties to the patient-physician relationship and how their interests might affect the obligations of physicians. Many physicians would applaud our traditional focus, for they believe that acting in the best interests of patients, and not those of third parties, is the physician's *sole* primary obligation. Moreover, our two models tend to support the World Medical Association's principle that "The health of my patient will be my first consideration."[1] These considerations tempt us to take the following principle as axiomatic in medical ethics: Because the patient's medical needs come first, there can be no primary competing responsibility to a third party. Dr. Arnold Relman, editor of the *New England Journal of Medicine*, defends this principle in the following form: "A physician's obligation is primarily to help his patient, and *not* the patient's parents or next of kin or legal guardian."[2]

The rule that the patient always comes first has undoubted intuitive appeal, as well as the weight of medical tradition. On closer examination, however, this principle rests on the dubious, indeed indefensible, assumption that the patient-physician relationship never involves primary obligations to third parties. The physician's professional relationships are multileveled. It is not uncommon for a physician's initial contact with a patient to come through a third party, and the relationship may encompass several other levels. For example, a woman may request health care services from the family physician for her seriously ill husband. After examining the patient and assessing his needs, the physician in turn may contact a local visiting nurse, who visits the home to provide required services. In

[1]World Medical Association, "Declaration of Geneva," *World Medical Association Bulletin*, 1, (3 July 1949): 109.

[2]"Treating Children Without Parental Consent," in *Troubling Problems in Medical Ethics*, ed. M. Basson (New York: Allen Liss, 1981), p. 109.

.addition, the physician's fees, as well as those of the nurse, are often paid by third parties. Private insurance, health maintenance organizations, and publicly funded programs such as Medicare and Medicaid may place restrictions on payment for certain services.

There are compelling moral reasons why the physician must consider the interests of such third parties. For example, third parties such as spouses, parents, and guardians often have rights and responsibilities that cannot be ignored. They may be the patient's fiduciary no less than the physician, and they may have legal authority to act to benefit the patient. At the same time, these parties may be significantly harmed if the physician acts in the best interests of the patient alone. The parents of a seriously ill infant may, for example, suffer overwhelming emotional, psychological, and financial consequences if their child is aggressively treated.[3]

Third parties also shape the physician's responsibilities because of the many roles the physician plays in contemporary medicine, particularly institutional roles. For example, the physician may be a research investigator or have public health responsibilities. Promoting the best interests of a patient—under the directives of the beneficence and autonomy models—may threaten or even harm the best interests of others the physician is expected to serve in these roles—for example, future patients and the local community. In these circumstances the general philosophical *principle* of beneficence (though not the beneficence *model*) directs the physician to promote the interests of third parties,[4] and this may generate obligations that conflict with or even override the physician's obligations to a patient.

Because they focus exclusively on the best interests of patients, the beneficence and autonomy models of moral responsibility in medicine are, by themselves, unable to take into account such obligations to third parties. At most, the two models have the moral power to determine that the physician must, *as a prima facie duty,* put the patient's best interests first. They do not tell the physician how to weigh the requirements of the models against a competing principle that would put some third party's best interests first. There is, therefore, no *a priori* ground for asserting that third-party obligations cannot be primary.

As a consequence, we argue in this chapter that "The health of my patient will be my first consideration" is but *one* prima facie valid principle. It must yield on occasion to a more complex account of conflicts between obli-

---

[3]See Natalie Abrams, "Scope of Beneficence in Health Care," in *Beneficence and Health Care,* ed. Earl Shelp (Boston: D. Reidel, 1982), p. 194. For a compelling account of these issues from the parental perspective, see Robert and Peggy Stinson, *The Long Dying of Baby Andrew* (Boston: Atlantic–Little, Brown, 1983).

[4]Others have analyzed the physician's moral conflict differently. Robert Veatch, for example, insists on a lexical order that places a principle of justice over that of beneficence. This leads him to a quite different account of how conflicts based in third-party interests might be resolved. See his *A Theory of Medical Ethics* (New York: Basic Books, 1982), Chapters 6, 12, and 13.

gations to patients and obligations to third parties. We shall see in this chapter that these conflicts are resolvable in one of three ways: (1) In some instances obligations to patients justifiably override those to third parties. (2) In other instances the obligations owed to patients and third parties are equal in weight, and the physician faces a genuine moral dilemma—that is, a circumstance involving a conflict of obligations, where inevitably an outcome of great value will be lost by pursuing one obligation at the expense of another. (3) Finally, in still other cases, the weight of morality shifts in favor of third-party interests, and obligations owed to third parties override those owed to patients.

We divide our discussion of third-party interests into two sections. In the first we address the physician's obligations to those in a fiduciary relationship with the patient. We consider, in particular, the physician's obligations to parents and guardians. In the second section we examine the physician's role-related obligations to certain other third parties, in particular, to health care institutions, educational and research institutions and their objectives, the patient's employer, and the local community and state. We do not claim that these categories exhaustively cover relevant third parties,[5] but there can be little doubt that the interests of these parties commonly create moral conflicts for many physicians and that these conflicts have received insufficient attention in both medicine and medical ethics.[6]

THIRD PARTIES WITH FIDUCIARY OBLIGATIONS: PARENTS AND GUARDIANS

We begin with an analysis of the physician's conflicting obligations to patients and to their fiduciaries—in particular, parents and guardians. A physician must sometimes abide by the decisions of parents and guardians, and sometimes must accept them even if he or she believes the decisions are not in the best interests of the child. Indeed, some have argued that the *child* is the third party in such circumstances, because the physician's contract is with the fiduciary parents, a view we reject.[7] Such a context is rife with the

---

[5]See, for example, H. Kuschner, "The Homosexual Husband and Physician Confidentiality," *Hastings Center Report* 7 (April 1977): 15–17, and Kim Marie Thorburn, "Croaker's Dilemma: Should Prison Physicians Serve Prisons or Prisoners?" *Western Journal of Medicine* 134 (May 1981): 457–61, for two problems that do not fit any of our categories.

[6]In a study of how physicians reason about critically ill patients, Diana Crane concludes that "Very few doctors seemed to have given such matters enough consideration to have worked out a philosophical position toward them." *The Sanctity of Social Life: Physicians' Treatment of Critically Ill Patients* (New York: Russell Sage Foundation, 1975), p. 76.

[7]In "Involuntary Euthanasia of Defective Newborns: A Legal Analysis," *Stanford Law Review* 27 (1975), John Robertson argues that the infant is effectively a third-party beneficiary by virtue of the parents' contract with the physicians.

potential for moral conflict. For example, parents sometimes make poor and even disastrous decisions for children, including circumstances of neglect and unjustified decisions to allow newborn infants to die. But the reverse may also be true: Adolescents may make disastrous decisions that they wish to shield from their parents—for example, decisions about sexual activity that eventuate in a need for medical care. The physician can have powerful obligations to both parents and children in such circumstances and may be trapped between competing obligations. As one court recently put it, there can be agonizing conflict between the "parental rights doctrine" and the "doctrine of the best interests of the child."[8]

We narrow our investigation here to conflicts involving the treatment of life-threatening conditions of infants and conflicts involving the control of confidential information about adolescent minors in sexual matters. Because the fiduciary—the parent or guardian—is expected to act to benefit the patient, we shall consider the obligations of the parent or guardian to protect the patient as well as the potential harm that may result if those obligations are discharged in certain ways. Our goal in each case is to determine whether the physician's obligations to avoid harm to the patient or to respect the rights of the patient outweigh conflicting obligations to avoid harm to the fiduciary or to respect the rights of the fiduciary.

Children with Life-Threatening Conditions

Raymond Duff and A. G. M. Campbell have reported that fourteen percent of the deaths recorded in the special-care nursery of the Yale–New Haven Hospital from January 1, 1970 through June 30, 1972, were associated with refusal, withholding, discontinuance, or withdrawal of treatment. The parents' decision was usually the decisive consideration, and Drs. Duff and Campbell view these parental decisions as generally legitimate.[9] By contrast, some institutions, such as Children's Hospital in Philadelphia, have a reputation for being much more aggressive.[10] They rarely discontinue or withhold treatment, irrespective of parental desires. Despite variations from institution to institution and physician to physician,

---

[8]*Guardianship of Becker,* Superior Court of Santa Clara, California, 1981, no. 101981, p. 1. This wardship case involves a Down's child with an at-birth ventricular septal defect of the heart and possible need for life-prolonging surgery. The court asserts that the case has "floundered on the rock of parental rights." But see note 50, which asserts grounds for overriding these rights.

[9]R. S. Duff and A. G. M. Campbell, "Moral and Ethical Dilemmas in the Special Care Nursery," *The New England Journal of Medicine* 289 (1973): 890–94. See also "On Deciding the Care of Severely Handicapped or Dying Persons with Particular Reference to Infants," *Pediatrics* 57 (1976): 487–93; and "Counselling Families and Deciding Care of Severely Defective Children," *Pediatrics* 67 (1981): 315–20. This perspective has clearly been influential in American medicine. See *Current Opinions of the Judicial Council of the A.M.A.,* Article 2. 10 (Chicago: American Medical Association, 1982).

[10]See D. C. Drake, "Keeping Infants Alive Is Only Half the Battle," *Philadelphia Inquirer* (September 24, 1978): 16.

questions remain about how the physician should respond if parents refuse permission for treatment of their seriously ill infant. This is but one instance of the more general problem of how the physician should weigh the interests of parents in determining his or her moral responsibilities. As we saw in chapter one, these matters are increasing in complexity because various governmental bodies—courts, legislatures, and regulatory agencies—are now more actively involved.

We begin our analysis with the following case: A baby girl is born with trisomy 21 (Down's syndrome), a genetic defect that involves varying and, at birth, unpredictable levels of mental retardation. The baby also has a life-threatening defect, an esophogeal-tracheal fistula, an opening between the baby's airway and passage to the stomach. The danger of this anatomical malformation is that her lungs can become infected or even blocked as a result of contact with food regurgitated from her stomach into her lungs. As a consequence, this infant cannot be fed by mouth. If the defect is not corrected by surgical intervention to close the opening, or if the baby is not supplied with nutrients by artificial means, she will die by dehydration. In addition, if her anatomical malformation is not corrected, she is at risk of contracting aspiration pneumonia, which, if not treated, will take her life— probably before dehydration. The parents, George and Sandra Breckner, already have three children, ages two, five, and seven. Together they earn a moderate wage. They refuse treatment on the grounds that it would not be worth the effort and ultimate costs—neither for the child's sake nor for theirs. The baby will be mentally retarded, they note, and raising a handicapped child would impose psychological, emotional, and serious financial burdens on them and their other children.

We argued in chapter five (p. 131) that the beneficence model is the basis for the physician's responsibility for this range of patients. Because this patient is irreversibly nonautonomous and has no value history, the third guide to intervention applies. The beneficence model, which is the basis for this guide, establishes an obligation to treat baby girl Breckner. Doing so avoids premature death and makes it possible to ameliorate her mental handicap. But should the physician simply abide by the dictates of the beneficence model, as if there were no obligations to the Breckners?

One approach to this question is to examine the answers given by physicians themselves. A national survey of pediatricians and pediatric surgeons presented questions on ethical issues such as those raised by the baby girl Breckner case. The results indicate that many physicians take quite seriously, and the majority take *most* seriously, the interests and expressed preferences of parents.[11] In many circumstances they believe it is permissi-

[11]Anthony Shaw, Judson G. Randolph, and Barbara Manard, "Ethical Issues in Pediatric Surgery: A National Survey of Pediatricians and Pediatric Surgeons," *Pediatrics* 60 (suppl., 1977): 588–99. For similar attitudes among British physicians, see the testimony in *In re* B (A Minor). 7 August 1981, in *The Weekly Law Reports* (27 November 1981): 1423.

ble for parents and physicians to make a joint decision to allow an infant to die. Of the surgeons polled, 76.8 percent reported that they would "acquiesce in parents' decisions" for nontreatment. The infant's "potential quality of life" was listed as the first or second criterion for justifying a decision by 90.7 percent of pediatric surgeons and by 86.3 percent of pediatricians. However, 49.8 percent of pediatric surgeons and 40.0 percent of pediatricians listed "possible adverse effects on the family" as the first or second criterion in making such a decision.[12] When asked generally about factors that influence the management of patients like baby girl Breckner, pediatric surgeons listed the infant's family as their first concern, while pediatricians listed it as their second, their primary concern being the infant.

This ambivalence is consistent with historical views about treatment of seriously ill infants. On the one hand, a prominent thesis has been that failure to treat such infants is unjustified because they are persons with a full set of legal rights.[13] On the other hand, there has been a wide tolerance of the failure to treat these infants, even a toleration of their being killed by their parents.[14] However, neither historical practices nor attitudes and polls about preferences constitute philosophical argument. In the end they do not provide a satisfactory answer for this question: In what respects, if any, do the interests of parents (and perhaps other family members) determine the physician's obligations in cases like that of baby girl Breckner?

To answer this question, we first need an understanding of parental obligations and interests. What obligations do Mr. and Mrs. Breckner have regarding the treatment of their infant? Are they morally free to refuse treatment for any reason they regard as sufficient? To the latter question the answer is decisively negative. From the legal as well as the moral point of view, the responsibility of parents toward their children is defined as that of the fiduciary: They are to act in the best interests of the child. While the common-law tradition treats children as chattels (personal property) of their parents, owing obedience to their dictates about education and medical intervention, it is also assumed in law that parents, as fiduciaries, always

[12]Ibid., 596, 593. These results are largely corroborated in I. David Todres et al., "Pediatricians' Attitudes Affecting Decision-Making in Defective Newborns," *Pediatrics* 60 (1977): 197–201.

[13]John Beck, *An Inaugural Dissertation on Infanticide* (New York: J. Seymour, 1817). For a more recent statement, see the articles by Robertson and Fost (note 15) and T. S. Ellis, "Letting Defective Babies Die: Who Decides?" *American Journal of Law and Medicine* 7 (1982): 393–423.

[14]For a classical description of different cultural attitudes about infanticide, see Edward A. Westermarck, "The Killing of Parents, Sick Persons, Children—Feticide," in his *The Origin and Development of the Moral Ideas* (London: Macmillan and Co., 1906–1908), vol. 1, chap. 17, pp. 393–413. See also Lloyd DeMause, ed., *The History of Childhood* (New York: Psychohistory Press, 1974).

act in their children's best interests. The state is not to interfere until it and the parents disagree regarding some decision with potentially serious consequences for the child. For this reason, the state—which has fiduciary responsibilities it may assert in a petition for guardianship—has often intervened in cases like that presented by the Breckner baby.

The state traditionally has had the right to seize authority to act in the best interests of children, and incompetents generally, in order to protect them from serious harm that parents or guardians might cause or permit.[15] When the best interests test is applied by the courts to the parent as decisionmaker, the test sometimes has been treated in a highly malleable fashion, taking into account intangible factors of questionable importance. For example, in cases where parents seek court permission for a kidney transplant from an incompetent minor to a competent sibling, the best interests of the donor have occasionally taken into account projected psychological trauma resulting from the death of the sibling and psychological benefits of the unselfish act of donation.[16] Consideration of such factors can easily lead to abuse, and the safest application of the best interests standard should require reference to *tangible* factors, such as demonstrable and significant physical, financial, and psychological risks.

The Breckners, then, are bound by certain obligations that constitute the parental role, namely to see to it that their daughter's best interests are promoted by her physicians. Following the principle of beneficence (not, of course, the beneficence model), and assuming normal circumstances, their obligation is to authorize the required surgery. The obligations of the Breckners and the attending physicians coincide in protecting their daughter's best interests through vigorous medical intervention. Accordingly, it seems reasonably clear that this child's interests in medical treatment ought to override the interests of the parents, and if the parents reach an unacceptable decision, the physician should attempt to overrule it. The physician's obligation in such cases is primarily to the patient. However, this conclusion can be escaped if it is genuinely in the best interests of the child *not* to have the surgery, as it is in some cases of very severe abnormalities and problems. This could be the case if the treatment is futile

---

[15]Every state in the U.S. requires parents to provide necessary medical assistance, and any failure to do so that causes death may result in prosecution for manslaughter or murder. Many forms of medical neglect may result in criminal charges. A physician who accepts such a parental decision may also be criminally liable, because he or she, too, has breached a legal duty of care. See John A. Robertson and Norman Fost, "Passive Euthanasia of Defective Newborn Infants: Legal Considerations," *Journal of Pediatrics* 88 (1976): 883–89.

[16]The precedent case for many later cases is *Strunk v. Strunk*, 445 S.W.2d 145 (Ky. 1969). See also *Hart v. Brown*, 289 A2d 386 (Conn. 1972). Contrast *Lausier v. Pescinski*, 67 Wis. 2d 4, 226 N.W.2d 180 (1975). See also John A. Robertson, "Organ Donations by Incompetents and the Substituted Judgment Doctrine," *Columbia Law Review* 76 (1976), esp. pp. 57–65.

because death is imminent or the patient is irreversibly dying, or if the burdens of treatment clearly outweigh the benefits to the patient.[17]

When it comes to the question of whether, after she has recovered from the surgery and is in stable condition, baby girl Breckner should go home, be placed in foster care, be institutionalized, or be placed for adoption, the moral weight of other parental interests may increase. The psychological, emotional, and financial burdens of raising a handicapped child, while giving their other children the basic attention they require, could well prove catastrophic for the Breckners. They may, therefore, have legitimate reasons for placing their daughter in an institution. However, this course may not be in their baby's best interests because institutionalized mentally retarded children do not always show the same progress as mentally retarded children raised at home.[18] An institution *could* theoretically provide satisfactory treatment, and the baby's welfare could be validly weighed against other considerations of family welfare—a delicate but often inescapable tradeoff.

If the Breckners ask the physician to help them make arrangements for their child to be institutionalized, the physician may face a tragic dilemma. Acting on such a request could worsen the child's treatment and inhibit development, while declining to act on the request could create significant burdens for the parents, perhaps resulting in severe stress for other children or for the marriage.[19] The beneficence model, applied to the patient, and the principle of beneficence, applied to the parents (and their children), may reveal that an equal moral weight is attached to each alternative.

[17]These justifying conditions are explored in detail in Tom L. Beauchamp and James Childress, *Principles of Biomedical Ethics*, 2d ed. (New York: Oxford University Press, 1983), Chapter 4. For important related arguments, see Terrence F. Ackerman, "Meningomyelocele and Parental Commitment: A Policy Proposal Regarding Selection for Treatment," *Man and Medicine* 5 (1980): 291ff.; "The Limits of Beneficence," *Hastings Center Report* 10 (August 1980): 13–18; Albert R. Jonsen and Michael J. Garland, "A Moral Policy for Life/Death Decisions in the Intensive Care Nursery," in *Ethics of Newborn Intensive Care*, ed. Albert R. Jonsen and Michael J. Garland (Berkeley: University of California, Institute of Governmental Studies, 1976); H. Tristram Engelhardt, Jr., "Ethical Issues in Aiding the Death of Young Children," in *Beneficent Euthanasia*, ed. Marvin Kohl (Buffalo, N.Y.: Prometheus Books, 1975); R. B. Zachary, "Ethical and Social Aspects of Treatment of Spina Bifida," *Lancet* 2 (3 August 1968): 274–76; John M. Freeman, "To Treat or Not to Treat: Ethical Dilemmas of Treating the Infant with a Myelomeningocele," *Clinical Neurosurgery* 20 (1973): 134–46; John Lorber, "Selective Treatment of Myelomeningocele: To Treat or Not to Treat?" *Pediatrics* 53 (1974): 307–8; several articles in Chester Swinyard, ed., *Decision Making and the Defective Newborn* (Springfield, Ill.: Charles C Thomas, 1978); and President's Commission for the Study of Ethical Problems in Medicine and Biomedical and Behavioral Research, *Deciding to Forego Life-Sustaining Treatment* (Washington, D.C.: U.S. Government Printing Office, 1983), pp. 6–8 and 197–229. These problems are often discussed in law and ethics alike in terms of the confusing distinction between withholding ordinary means and withholding extraordinary means.

[18]Robert B. Edgerton, *Mental Retardation* (Cambridge: Harvard University Press, 1979), especially p. 38ff.

[19]See G. M. Hunt, "Implications of the Treatment of Myelomeningocele for the Child and His Family," *Lancet* 2 (1973): 1308–10; and E. H. Hare et al., "Spina Bifida Cystica and Family Stress," *British Medical Journal* 2 (24 September 1966): 757–60.

If such a dilemma arises, the ideal of putting the patient's interest first may still be of some help to the physician, who might ask the Breckners to reconsider, especially in light of the impact that alternatives like institutionalization may have on their daughter. This alternative, however, will not always be available.

It is not hard to imagine modestly different cases in which the interests of parents may be overriding. Suppose, for example, that Mr. Breckner is deeply disturbed by the fact that his daughter is handicapped, so disturbed that he is near the psychological breaking point. This problem has led to several conflicts and arguments with his supervisors at work, and he has been threatened with dismissal. The other children, Mrs. Breckner reports, have asked, "What's wrong with Daddy?" She adds that she is afraid that her husband might lose his job. In such circumstances, the burdens of bringing the baby home may prove intolerable to Mr. Breckner, with disastrous consequences for the health and general well-being of his wife and other children and the financial base of the family. The physician may then have an obligation to facilitate the request for institutionalization, based on Mr. Breckner's best interests and the family's best interests.[20] This obligation overrides the physician's obligation to promote the infant's best interests, which are reasonably predicted to be compromised by institutionalization. To protect the infant's interests in situations such as this, physicians rightly seek alternatives such as foster care, while distressed parents receive counseling and reassess their ability to bring their child home. In some circumstances—usually those in which the infant is profoundly and/or multiply handicapped—the demands of infant care can exceed the resources of almost any family. It is then clearly justified, under the principle of beneficence, for the physician to recommend and arrange alternative care, even if the infant's best interests are compromised by doing so.

In sum, we have seen in this section that in cases involving life-threatening conditions of children the physician faces conflicting obligations. In those cases in which it is in the patient's best interests to be treated, parents usually have an obligation to authorize treatment, an obligation that tends to override personal interests they might have. In such circumstances, the "weight of morality" resides with the normal obligation of the physician to provide treatment. We also saw that decisions for or against treatment are not the whole of the matter in cases involving life-threatening conditions. If treatment is provided, other obligations may

---

[20]It also seems clear that, based on the principle of beneficence, the physician has an obligation to offer or to recommend counseling to Mr. Breckner. On this topic, see Norman Fost, "Counseling Families Who Have a Child with a Severe Congenital Anomaly," *Pediatrics* 67 (March 1981): 321–24. For a compelling study of the reaction of parents to children with serious birth defects, see Rosalyn Benjamin Darling, *Families Against Society: A Study of Reactions to Children with Birth Defects* (Beverly Hills, Calif.: Sage Publications, 1979).

have to be determined, especially regarding the continued care and support of the child. The physician faces genuine dilemmas, in some cases between obligations to the child and obligations to parents, and in still other cases the obligations to parents justifiably override what the physician recognizes to be the patient's best interests.

Adolescent Sexuality and Privacy

Conflicts between the patient's interests and those of the parents increase in complexity when older children are involved. In recent years older children have ever more frequently been recognized as developing in autonomy and not as mere chattels of their parents (or the state, in the case of wards). These children are now acknowledged as having legal and moral rights (and responsibilities) unimagined in earlier times. There is currently a legal trend toward the explication and expansion of children's rights, some of which are referred to as "rights of self-determination." Similarly, many child psychologists view autonomy on a sliding scale from no autonomy to more or less full autonomy, as the child develops from birth to late adolescence.[21] The problem is how full an older child's autonomy must be before the child's decisions and the obligations they create override obligations to respect the decisions of their parents or guardians.

This problem is especially difficult in cases where minor children seek medical treatment without their parents' knowledge or consent. Ordinarily, parental decisions for the benefit of their children require access to information in the sole possession of their children's physician. Obligations to maintain a very young child's confidentiality are usually not given overriding authority, but as autonomy grows in presence and importance, obligations to maintain the child's privacy and confidentiality also increase in weight.

These autonomy-based considerations are given additional weight from the perspective of the beneficence model. Irresponsible parents—for example, those who drink heavily and abuse the child—create grounds for protecting the child's confidentiality that are not otherwise present. Also, young people may not trust the physician without assurances of confidentiality. With such assurances, the adolescent patient is more likely to be open and honest, a key condition in the pursuit of the goods highlighted in the beneficence model. These reasons underlie laws in virtually every state in the U.S. allowing physicians to treat venereal disease in adolescents without parental consent.[22] At some point, the parent loses all rights of special access. But at what point?

---

[21]See Lucy Rau Ferguson, "The Competence and Freedom of Children to Make Choices Regarding Participation in Biomedical and Behavioral Research," in *Research Involving Children, Appendix* (Washington, D.C.: DHHS for the National Commission for the Protection of Human Subjects, 1977), pp. 4–1 to 4–42.

[22]See H. F. Pilpel, "Minors' Rights to Medical Care," *Albany Law Review* 36 (1972): 462ff.

Leading cases emerged in *Planned Parenthood of Central Missouri v. Danforth* and *Bellotti v. Baird*,[23] where the United States Supreme Court invalidated state statutes requiring parental consent, consultation, or notification in cases of abortions for minors. The Court ruled that the statutes were impermissible because they restricted the *competent* minor's constitutional rights of privacy and imposed an undue burden on the right to seek an abortion. The Court, however, did not set out a relevant test for "competence"—a major consideration, especially if legal and moral demands of informed consent are pertinent. (See chapters three and five.) Other medical interventions that some minors may request without parental consent include treatment for venereal disease, addiction, pregnancy, consultation for contraception, treatment for psychological disturbance, blood donation, treatment for emergency, "necessary services," and treatment for reportable disease. Legal accessibility to these treatments varies from state to state, and moral views are no less settled than the legal situation.

If *Danforth* and *Bellotti* were accepted as the final word, one might be tempted to draw the following conclusion: In the case of adolescents and their autonomous decisions about their own sexuality (not merely a choice for abortion), "Put the patient's interests first" is an absolute principle, one that in every case overrides the principle that the parents' interests in their child should come first. This view is consistent with the demands of both models, which seem to converge on a strong obligation of confidentiality. It is not difficult, however, to imagine circumstances in which this obligation of confidentiality to the adolescent patient is weaker. This obligation would clearly be weakened if a profound threat to health or life were present, but it would be weakened in less dramatic cases as well.

Suppose that an adolescent requesting an abortion is deeply and perhaps irrationally fearful of her parents' possibly negative reaction to her decision. The physician may detect that the patient in these circumstances takes this view primarily because of the views of her friends and not because she has made a thoughtful assessment of her parents' likely response. In addition, the physician may know her parents and have good reason to believe that while they would not necessarily accept her choice or the values it expresses, they would be concerned to help her reach an autonomous decision. If her parents are excluded from helping her reach a thoughtful decision, the relationship between them may be damaged, especially if the parents discover the truth later. In short, the patient's choice for an abortion may reflect a degree of reduced autonomy, her parents might be an invaluable resource for an autonomous decision, and her parents might be harmed by being excluded.

---

[23]*Planned Parenthood of Central Missouri v. Danforth*, 428 U.S. 52 (1976) and *Bellotti v. Baird*, 443 U.S. 622 (1979). See also *Carey v. Population Services Int'l.*, 431 U.S. 678 (1977)—a contraception case—and contrast *H.L. v. Matheson*, 101 S.Ct. 1164 (1981) to all three of the above.

Because the interests of the parents coincide with the patient's best interest, it would be unreasonable to exclude her parents altogether. To be sure, including them might unduly influence the patient, and in such circumstances the physician might be faced with a genuine dilemma. However, consider the following case: The young woman's parents know that she is pregnant. She believes that they want her to have an abortion, but the physician has spoken with them and knows that they do not. The young woman very much wants to keep her baby and tells the physician that she thinks her parents do not understand her at all and are wrong and insensitive to want her to have an abortion. In the physician's judgment, the patient's growing bitterness and anger toward her parents could severely damage an otherwise positive relationship with them. The only way to avoid damaging the relationship irreparably would be to involve the parents in the patient's decisions about her pregnancy, even if she did not believe that doing so would be in her best interests.[24]

The physician, then, must carefully weigh all competing obligations when dealing with conflicts between obligations to minors who are patients and obligations to their parents. Broad declarations of parents' rights or of children's rights do a disservice, rather than a service, and may unnecessarily squeeze the physician into an untenable position. Distinctive virtues such as compassion or tact may serve the physician more steadily than moral principles of duty or assertions of rights. If the adolescent's confidentiality merits rigid protection, considerable tact and compassion may be demanded, because the physician may have to deflect well-intended—and very direct—parental inquiries concerning the source and nature of the child's problem.

THIRD PARTIES WITH NONFIDUCIARY OBLIGATIONS

The physician has potentially conflicting obligations to third parties other than fiduciaries such as parents and guardians. Some of these third parties—e.g., health care institutions and employers—may have some limited fiduciary obligations to the patient. But they also have competing obligations and interests. Unlike parents, whose *primary* charge is to act as the patient's fiduciary, these third parties have primary responsibilities that are sometimes remote from serving the patient's interests. In this section we explore how the physician should weigh obligations based in such interests.

---

[24]A convincing case of an 11-year-old girl whose confidentiality about venereal disease was not broken, but probably should have been, is found in Norman Fost, "Ethical Problems in Pediatrics," *Current Problems in Pediatrics* 6 (October 1976): 25. Fost argues that "an unnecessary and often harmful isolation from the parents" can be created by rules of confidentiality.

Health Care Institutions

Physicians practice ever less frequently in the solo style of one patient–one physician. Increasingly, they provide care to patients in institutional settings such as group practices, clinics, health maintenance organizations (HMOs), private (nonprofit and profit) hospitals, nursing homes, and hospices. In a group practice, for example, a patient is seen primarily by one physician but also, on occasion, by other physicians in the group, especially in multi-specialty group practices. In clinics and HMOs the physician practices alongside many health care professionals, and in hospitals the patient is seen and treated by a sometimes bewildering train of physicians, nurses, and other health care professionals, including medical students and physicians in training. As the number of highly specialized practitioners increases, the individual responsibilities they have for patients tend to decrease. Sometimes the patient may not have a single physician in charge of the case—and no one to turn to for information and comfort.

The institutional organization of medical care has expanded in novel directions in order to provide a quantity and quality of care that the individual physician cannot provide.[25] While health care institutions are committed to the well-being of patients, their large scale and complexity generate commitments to other values as well. These tend to cluster around considerations of efficiency, with special emphasis on cost-effectiveness and cost-reduction, and, increasingly, profit. Goods and harms understood from the perspective of medicine can conflict with broader, though related, institutional perspectives. The patient, too, may not accept such an institutional perspective, and this produces conflicts between obligations based in beneficence generally and obligations based in the autonomy model. The following cases illustrate these conflicts.

Case Study: Cost Effectiveness and Restricting a Patient's Access to Medication. Samuel Browning, a forty-six-year-old civil engineer, presents to his physician in his health maintenance organization with an upper respiratory tract infection. The physician explains to Mr. Browning that, because his infection is probably viral in nature, antibiotic medication will not be useful in combating it. The physician explains that the HMO has adopted the cost-saving policy of not prescribing such medication unless the patient also has a bacterial infection. Mr. Browning insists, nonetheless, that he would like to have a prescription for antibiotics, on the chance that there may be a bacterial infection, which would clear up more quickly with such medication.

The (hypothetical) institutional policy in this case has a powerful rationale. As a result of excessive reliance on antibiotics, bacteria have not only

---

[25]For an important analysis of the impact of the institutionalization of medicine, see Paul Starr, *The Social Transformation of American Medicine* (New York: Basic Books, 1982).

not been eliminated from the environment, they have begun to mutate in response to exposure to the wide range of antibiotics now in use. The result is that new, more resilient bacteria have evolved. Some bacterial infections now require heavy doses of potent antibiotics, thus creating significant risks from the medication itself. Mutation of bacteria can also take place in an individual over time. Hence, at both the population and individual levels, excessive use of antibiotics poses new health risks.

Because the use of antibiotics in the treatment of viral upper respiratory infections has been identified as a factor in the excessive use of antibiotics, there have been proposals in the medical community to use them only when there is evidence that the patient has a bacterial infection. Viral infections of the upper respiratory tract are usually self-limiting, and bacterial infections do not always accompany such infections. As a rule there is no need to prescribe antibiotics for routine instances of the disease unless laboratory tests confirm the presence of a bacterial infection. According to the beneficence model, therefore, prescribing antibiotics to patients without bacterial infections exposes them to unnecesary risks, and the physician has an obligation not to do so.

The HMO to which Mr. Browning belongs, which is also the employer of his physician, provides a $2.00 deductible for prescriptions: A patient pays $2.00 for his or her prescription, with the HMO absorbing the balance of the cost. The HMO is funded by a prepayment mechanism, with subscribers' fees met in part by the subscriber and in part by his or her employer. The HMO has a fixed budget based on the total number of its subscribers, and it must deliver health care services to its subscribers without exhausting its budget. Cost-efficiency is thus a primary value. If cost reduction is consistent with satisfaction of the health care needs of subscribers, HMOs have an incentive to accomplish this goal. By not making prescriptions available for patients like Mr. Browning—unless there is a confirmed bacterial infection—significant cost reductions can be effected, while the patient's risks of morbidity will not be increased to an unacceptable level. A conflict of this sort between a patient's explicit request for medication and an HMO policy can easily be resolved from the physician's perspective. The physician's institutional obligations of cost-effective delivery of care do not *conflict* with obligations to serve the patient's best interests, as these are understood in the beneficence model. This happy resolution, however, is not the outcome in every such case.

Case Study: Resource Allocation for Intensive Newborn Care. Michael Brown was born in a community hospital in a normal delivery. Shortly after his birth, it was discovered that most of his small intestine was dead tissue and would have to be removed to save his life. He was rushed to a private hospital where the required surgery was performed. The surgeons had explained beforehand that this procedure might leave him with a portion of his small intestine too short for survival unless artificial feeding was administered for the rest of his life. He was subsequently placed on hyperalimentation (the direct supply of nutrients into the blood stream)—a very expensive form of treatment. Michael began to develop as a normal baby, though somewhat slowly. Both of his parents were unemployed and had no health insurance. By the time Michael had reached the age of six months, his hospital bill had reached $275,000, which the hospital absorbed. The hospital administrator at this point recommended to the board of trustees that, given the projected expenses of his care, Michael be released from the hospital and transferred to a state institution. He emphasized that the hospital had an obligation to provide care in charity cases, but he argued that the expense in Michael's case would be so excessive that the hospital's ability to meet the need of other indigent patients would be seriously threatened. He reported that the state institution would most likely not pay for the cost of hyperalimentation and that, without this treatment, Michael would die within ten to fifteen days. Reluctantly, the board accepted the administrator's recommendation, and Michael's physician was instructed to release him to a state institution where the physician did not practice.

In these circumstances, Michael's physician faces an agonizing dilemma. On the one hand, with continued hyperalimentation Michael could continue to live and develop, though for how long is uncertain. Under the beneficence model, the physician has an obligation to sustain Michael's life, at least until it becomes clear that it is not in his best interests to do so. This point seems not yet to have been reached. The physician also has obligations to the hospital, which in turn has obligations to others to use its resources efficiently. The physician is thus trapped between several levels of commitments and loyalties. There is no tidy resolution of the sort presented in the HMO case. Moreover, we shall now see that there are situations in which the physician's obligation to a health care institution may justifiably override obligations to his or her patient.

Case Study: A Request for Plastic Surgery. Marcia Bloom's foot was injured ten years ago when a tree limb her husband was cutting fell on it. The surgical repair left what she has always regarded as ugly scars, and she tries to avoid wearing shoes that expose them. Two years ago, Mrs. Bloom joined an HMO to enjoy the reduced expenses of health care for her family. When she asks her HMO physician if plastic surgery to remove the scar tissue is included in the benefit package, she is told that it is not, because the disfigurement of her foot poses no serious health risks. She replies that she is self-conscious about the scarring and is sometimes depressed to the point of tears.

The conflict for the physician in this case is the following: Mrs. Bloom's condition is a source of genuine psychological distress, and the beneficence model would justify an obligation to remove the cause of this distress. Moreover, under the autonomy model, Mrs. Bloom's distress should be taken seriously by the physician because the patient takes the problem so seriously. The HMO, however, requires her physician to refuse her request, and all similar requests, as a cost-saving measure. In addition, the HMO physician knows that Mrs. Bloom, along with other subscribers with similar problems, implicitly agreed to such a restriction when she joined the HMO, and, while her interest is genuine in having the appearance of her foot improved, alternative measures are available to her, at lower costs to the HMO—e.g., psychological counseling. The patient's autonomy claims are minimal because of her implicit acceptance of a restricted range of benefits when she joined the HMO. Thus, while the physician's obligations to Mrs. Bloom under the beneficence model remain intact, they are overriden by the physician's obligation to carry out the HMO policy.[26] The justification for this conclusion rests on limited resources and the nature of the low-cost plan in which Mrs. Bloom has voluntarily enrolled: Those resources cannot be efficiently managed to meet the health care needs of all subscribers if all requests like Mrs. Bloom's are satisfied.

To summarize, in this section we have found a range of conflicts to be generated by third-party interests and claims of health care institutions on physicians: (1) conflicts resolvable in favor of the patient's best interests, (2) conflicts involving perhaps irresolvable dilemmas, and (3) conflicts that are resolvable in favor of the institution's interests.

While health care institutions are committed to patients who come to them for care, they also embrace other values that may compete with the interests of patients. This situation is generally unlike that of third-party interests of parents, which, because they are the interests of a fiduciary, are not as remote from the interests of their children as are interests like cost efficiency and cost-reduction.

Medical Research and Education

A major goal of medicine is to provide for medical care to future generations of patients by training physicians and by producing new knowledge, skills, medicines, and technologies. These enterprises, however, can be a source of conflict of obligations for clinicians engaged in both patient care and research or teaching.

Medical Research. Consider the role of the clinician-researcher. He or she has a dual responsibility that easily produces a conflict of obligations:

---

[26]Charles Fried has argued that if an institutional advantage can be gained for clients or patients that clearly promotes their best interests, it is professional negligence not to do so, even if the professional disapproves of the system's rules. A discussion of his point that relates specifically to medicine is found in Natalie Abrams, "Scope of Beneficence in Health Care," 196.

The physician is obligated to act in the patient's best interests and is also obligated to carry out research according to strict canons of scientific methodology. Controlled clinical trials require accurate confirmation of a scientific hypothesis. They can involve the random assignment of therapies and even placebos to patients, as well as other maneuvers intended to eliminate bias in the research. While in theory patients do not receive treatments that are known to be less safe or less effective than other available treatments, preliminary data occasionally indicate an increased efficacy of one therapy, and animal studies sometimes indicate efficacy prior to initiation of the trial.

In any event, it would be inconsistent with the beneficence model to *randomly* select a treatment for a patient *unless* he or she were involved in a clinical trial. As Arthur Schafer puts it, "regardless of whether a patient benefits from agreeing to become a research subject, the physician who attempts to combine the traditional role of healer with the modern role of scientist places himself in a situation that contains a potential conflict of values. His commitment can no longer be exclusively and unequivocally to promote the interests of his patients."[27] To preserve the integrity of the research protocol, physicians involved in clinical research would be obligated to make recommendations about care that the nonresearch physician would not make. How should the physician weight these competing obligations?

To illustrate these concerns, consider the following case. Gloria Wallace is an eighteen-year-old woman with Hodgkin's disease, a form of cancer. She is presently at stage II of the disease, for which the standard therapy is radiation. This treatment carries the risk of secondary cancer. An alternative treatment, still in the experimental stage, is "combined therapy": narrowly focused radiation (to reduce the secondary risk of cancer) combined with chemotherapy. The latter causes nausea and in some cases hair loss. Gloria's physician is part of a multisite research project that is examining the relative efficacy of this treatment, as compared with standard radiation treatment, in a randomized clinical trial. When presented with the information that she might receive combined therapy in the clinical trial if she should choose to participate in the project as a research subject, Gloria elects not to participate. Her reason is that she does not want to be disfigured.

If the role of the physician in this case is regarded as that of clinician alone, matters are unclouded: Ms. Wallace has been offered and has accepted the standard therapy. She has exercised her autonomy in an informed decision, which conforms to arguments in chapter three about the physician's obligation to obtain the informed decisions of patients. More-

---

[27]Arthur Schafer, "The Ethics of the Randomized Clinical Trial," *New England Journal of Medicine* 307 (16 September 1982): 720.

over, she has chosen a mode of treatment known to be effective for her disease. Thus, the physician's obligation to Ms. Wallace, based in both models of moral responsibility, is explicit. For the clinician who is also a research scientist, however, matters are more complex. The research in which Ms. Wallace is invited to participate is based on a morally justified goal—to develop for patients with her disease a form of therapy that possibly will reduce the risks of secondary cancer, while maintaining as much or greater efficacy in treating the disease than radiation alone.

This consideration is not irrelevant to the clinician's role: Without the new therapy, he or she will have no choice but to treat future patients by standard radiation therapy, which for some patients results in yet another form of cancer. The risk of secondary cancer is not eliminated with combined therapy, but it is hoped that its frequency will be reduced. When the two modes of treatment are viewed from the perspective of the beneficence model, the new, combined therapy—*if* shown to be as effective in combating the primary disease as the standard therapy—is the one that should be used, because it presents a lower level of risk. Here the dual roles of clinician and researcher produce a genuine moral dilemma. On the one hand, the physician as *clinician* is obligated to provide treatment that serves the patient's best interests, as directed by the beneficence and autonomy models. This obligation is most satisfactorily discharged by use of standard therapy because the experimental therapy has not yet been shown to be of equal or greater benefit. On the other hand, the principle of beneficence generates an obligation for the physician as *researcher* to benefit future patients with effective therapies that carry the lowest possible risks. The investigator also has institutional obligations to perform the research. He or she will not be able to discharge these obligations unless sufficient numbers of present patients participate in the experimental protocol. This might not occur if the physician were to act exclusively in the best interests of the patient. The physician in the dual role of clinician *and* researcher thus faces equally compelling claims on the part of present patients and those of future patients.[28]

Suppose, hypothetically, that the research program has begun to produce strong, but not yet conclusive, evidence that the combined therapy is more effective in causing remission than the standard therapy. The researcher may then experience pressure to bring as many patients as possible into the clinical trial, so that results can be validated expeditiously and the combined therapy can be more quickly accepted and introduced as the treatment of choice. Unlike the nonresearch physician, the research physician in these circumstances has an obligation to press forward vigorously to

---

[28]A similar problem is identified by D. Mark Mahler et al. regarding research on medical cost containment. See D. Mark Mahler, Robert M. Veatch, and Victor W. Seidel, "Ethical Issues in Informed Consent: Research on Medical Cost Containment," *Journal of the American Medical Association* 247 (22–29 January 1982): 481–85.

complete the study. Hence, he or she has a strong motivation to convince Ms. Wallace and his or her other patients with the disease to reconsider and join the research project as subjects for randomization. If Ms. Wallace's physician and clinician-researchers in cooperating sites simply accepted the refusals of patients like Ms. Wallace—who risk only hair loss or other temporary, reversible cosmetic changes—the research endeavor could be seriously impeded. In these circumstances, the interests of the third parties who will be benefited in the future by the new treatment, together with the institution's interests and objectives, become the overriding consideration for the researcher.

Medical Education. A similar range of conflicts is present in medical education. Patients who receive their medical care in clinics and hospitals that are teaching institutions are seen by medical students and physicians-in-training, as well as by practicing physicians. When so informed by their physician, some patients adamantly insist that they be examined and treated by their physician alone. Based on the autonomy model, it would seem that the physician's obligation is to respect the patient's wishes. The physician engaged in medical education, however, has the additional responsibility of assisting in the education of the next generation of physicians in order to serve the interests of future patients. If patients do not consent to be "teaching material" for students and others new to medical "practice," this important goal cannot be realized. The consequence might be that levels of care now enjoyed by patients will not be available to future patients. Thus, the academic physician faces a conflict of equally compelling interests: those of the patient presently in his or her care, and those of future patients who will be cared for by the students and physicians-in-training for whose education he or she also is responsible.

Consider the following case. Dr. Sean O'Malley is chief of cardiology in a university teaching hospital. In his educational role, Dr. O'Malley is responsible for the training of medical residents—physicians who have completed their medical degrees and are taking specialty training. Among the procedures that they must learn is how to thread a catheter (a hollow tube) into a patient's heart as part of a complex diagnostic procedure. This diagnostic intervention poses significant risk, even when performed by a physician with many years of experience. These risks increase if a relatively inexperienced resident performs the procedure. Dr. O'Malley is also the physician in charge of the care of patients who become "teaching material" for the residents. As the patient's physician, Dr. O'Malley would not be justified in placing the patient in a position where the risks involved when a resident performs catheterization fall below a minimally acceptable level of professional skill. As residents learn, incurring the possibility of such risk is inevitable. Yet if residents are not given the opportunity to learn, they will not be as competent to benefit future patients as they would be as the result of many such learning opportunities.

Ordinarily, this problem is handled by providing close supervision of physicians-in-training and medical students. At best, this approach reduces increased risk to the patients, but it does not always reduce risk to an acceptable minimum level.[29] Such risk is justifiably incurred, however, in the interests of future patients. If physicians are not provided with adequate training, they may well subject their patients to risks higher than those that present patients encounter at the hands of their physicians—an unacceptable balancing of goods and harms under the principle of beneficence. Obligations to such patients override those of present patients, who are themselves the beneficiaries of former teaching exercises on other patients.

Problems of Persuasion and Manipulation.   Institutional commitment to teaching and research facilities can also raise subtle questions about the limits of persuasion and manipulation as means to gain the cooperation of patients in medical research and education. Concerns about manipulation are of course ubiquitous in life—as testified by popular debates about whether or not various forms of advertising are manipulative. These are usually concerns about whether we are being played upon by devious or unfair techniques—whether or not that is the intention of the manipulator. Problems of manipulation and perhaps even coercion can be of importance in medicine because patients are often abnormally weak, dependent, and surrender-prone. Influences that can normally be resisted might become irresistible.

Dr. Franz Ingelfinger argued that "some element of coercion" is present in virtually every circumstance in which a physician asks a patient to join an experimental investigation. Ingelfinger characterized what he took to be a *typical* situation of influence as follows: "Incapacitated and hospitalized because of illness, frightened by strange and impersonal routines, and fearful for his health and perhaps life, the patient is far from exercising a free power of choice when the person to whom he anchors all his hopes asks, 'Say, you wouldn't mind, would you, if you joined some of the other patients on this floor and helped us to carry out some very important research we are doing?' . . . Here the thumb screws of coercion are . . . relentlessly applied . . . to the patient with disease."[30] The point to be extracted from such examples is that the physician could compel compliance both in education and in research by playing upon desperation, anxiety, boredom, hope, and a wide variety of human emotions so poignantly present in the

---

[29]For a moving account of how important it was to one leukemia patient to have the intravenous nurse-team draw blood, see Morris B. Abram, *The Day is Short* (New York: Harcourt Brace Jovanovich, 1982), p. 209.

[30]Franz J. Ingelfinger, "Informed (But Uneducated) Consent," *New England Journal of Medicine* 288 (31 August 1972): 465–66. See also Henry W. Riecken and Ruth Ravich, "Informed Consent to Biomedical Research in Veterans' Administration Hospitals," *Journal of the American Medical Association* 248 (16 July 1982): 344–48.

life of the hospitalized or seriously ill patient. Thus, what the physician regards as an attempt at truly rational persuasion may have the effect of irrational persuasion or manipulation because of the way in which the words tug at such patients' vulnerabilities.[31]

Education, advertising, and propaganda (to take some distant analogies) can certainly be used as rationally persuasive and quite acceptable techniques, but they can also easily glide into unjustifiable means of "persuasion," especially if a powerful authority figure employs them. Similarly, the influence of a physician may be welcomed by the patient and may be perfectly appropriate—up to a limiting point. Just as educators, advertising agencies, and propagandists can inadvertently (or advertently) move from persuasion to manipulation to coercion, so can physicians. It can be agonizingly difficult to pinpoint the conditions under which a surrender-prone patient, desperately needing an authority, willingly submits to the physician's authority, as distinct from the conditions under which a physician uses authority for undue, even exploitative, advantage.

It does not follow from these problems of medical practice that physicians *do* routinely manipulate or exploit the psychological vulnerabilities of patients. It follows only that patients are vulnerable to such forms of influence and that due care must be taken to cultivate virtues of restraint and compassion that avoid or minimize manipulation and coercion, especially in implementing obligations based on third-party interests in medical research and education.[32]

Employers

The third-party interests discussed thus far have generally not been altogether remote from those of serving the patient's interests. The patient's health and well-being are expectably at the forefront, even if they are not always foremost for health care, research, and academic institutions. Some third-party interests, however, diverge sharply from those of the patient. This is commonly the case in some dimensions of occupational medicine. For example, physicians who contract to examine job applicants or employees, physicians who are employed in industry, prisons, and the military to provide medical care for employees, or physicians who are employed to develop health-education and preventive-medicine programs regularly con-

---

[31]A complicating factor here—and elsewhere in medical practice—is conflict of interest for the physician. Thus, for example, the young clinical-researcher seeking tenure and other signs of recognition may allow ambition to override his or her moral responsibilities. The topic of conflicts of interests in medicine is a large one and, unfortunately, beyond the scope of this book.

[32]For concrete recommendations, see President's Commission for the Study of Ethical Problems in Medicine and Biomedical and Behavioral Research, *Making Health Care Decisions* (Washington, D.C.: U.S. Government Printing Office, 1982), Chapter 6, pp. 129–49.

front conflicts between the individual worker's best interests and the interests of an employer to whom the physician owes a contractual obligation.

The employer's best interests are not captured by the objectives of the beneficence model. Efficiency, cost-reduction, and profitability are among the employer's primary interests; maintaining the health and welfare of employees may often be a remote interest. The contract between physician and employer may, for example, require disclosure to the employer and records open to the company (and sometimes to unions). The occupational physician's obligation to disclose to employees the nature of health hazards that may exist in their workplace can be in direct conflict with these contractual commitments.

Case Study: Disclosing Health Hazards.   Dr. James Young is employed part time as medical director for a small company that produces cotton fabric in three mills employing about six hundred people. In response to recent reports about the connection between "brown lung" and high levels of cotton dust, the company has reduced the level of cotton dust in its mills by about twenty-five percent. The cost of additional reductions would result in the company's losing its already narrow competitive edge over imported fabrics. "Brown lung" is the common name for byssinosis, a form of chronic lung disease that in its severe form can be so debilitating that its victims cannot work and are often home-bound. Smokers have a larger risk of contracting the disease and of compounding its effects than do nonsmokers. Dr. Young estimates that at the present level of cotton dust in the mills, about twenty percent of the employees—both smokers and nonsmokers—may suffer some lung ailments, with about two percent of all employees—mostly smokers—actually contracting "brown lung." He submits a report to the company president with this information, together with his projections of employee risk. He recommends that the company consider initiating a campaign to inform employees of the risk of cotton dust, with special efforts to reach employees who smoke.

The president of the company, who is justifiably worried about the company's financial security, replies that such efforts would cause considerable disruption and undue anxiety, would be too expensive, and would inevitably affect productivity in the mills. He instructs Dr. Young to undertake no educational program. In this situation, the physician is caught in a conflict between an obligation to disclose health hazards to employees and an obligation to the employer. The company's competitive edge in the marketplace—upon which the employees' jobs all depend—is no small consideration, and from this perspective the company president is acting with good reason.

The Role of the Autonomy Model.   One way to understand the occupational physician's obligation to disclose hazards is in terms of the autonomy model, in particular, the right of employees to know about health hazards in the workplace. This obligation has emerged in recent years as a major issue in occupational health policy.[33] A general consensus has evolved that there is a right to know, and correlatively that there is a moral obligation on someone's part to disclose relevant information to workers. In 1980, the U.S. Occupational Safety and Health Administration (OSHA) promulgated federal regulations guaranteeing workers access to their medical and exposure records.[34] Legislation enacted in several states and cities lent further credibility to the claim that workers have a right to know. A New York state bill, for example, declares that employees and their representatives have a right to "*all* information relating to toxic substances"—a right that cannot be "waived as a condition of employment."[35] These developments are not entirely new to medicine. The "Code of Ethical Conduct for Physicians Providing Occupational Medical Services," for example, calls on member physicians to communicate health hazards "to individuals or groups potentially affected."[36]

There is, however, considerable ambiguity about which protections and actions workers' rights entail. The 1980 OSHA regulations established a strong worker right of *access* to information. With few exceptions, employers under this regulation are obligated to provide information within 15 days of receiving a request for access to medical records by an employee or an employee's designated representative. On its own initiative, an employer is obligated to inform workers first entering employment (and at least yearly thereafter) about the *existence* of medical and exposure records, the employee's rights of access to those records, and the person responsible for maintaining the records.[37] However, under the regulation, employers

[33]See Elihu D. Richter, "The Worker's Right to Know: Obstacles, Ambiguities, and Loopholes," *Journal of Health Politics, Policy and Law* 6 (1981): 340; Nicholas Ashford and Judith P. Katz, "Unsafe Working Conditions: Employee Rights Under the Labor Management Relations Act and the Occupational Safety and Health Act," *Notre Dame Lawyer* 52 (June 1977): 802–37; Gail Bronson, "Workers' Right to Know," *The Wall Street Journal* (Eastern Edition), 1 July 1977: 4 and Editorial, 1 January 1979; George Miller, "The Asbestos Coverup," *Congressional Record* (17 May 1979): E2363–64, and "Asbestos Health Hazards and Company Morality," *Congressional Record* (24 May 1979): E2523–24; NIOSH et al., "The Right to Know: Practical Problems and Policy Issues Arising from Exposure to Hazardous Chemical and Physical Agents in the Workplace," a report prepared at the request of the Subcommittee on Labor and the Committee on Human Resources, U.S. Senate (Washington, D.C.: July 1977); and Harold J. Magnuson, "The Right to Know," *Archives of Environmental Health* 32 (1977): 40–44.

[34]Occupational Safety and Health Administration, "Access to Employee Exposure and Medical Records—Final Rules," *Federal Register* (23 May 1980): 35212–77. (Hereafter referred to as OSHA regulations.) Future modifications in these regulations are a virtual certainty. An attempt at stringent revision was published in "Hazard Communication: Proposed Rules and Public Hearing Announcement," *Federal Register* (19 May 1982): 12092–124.

[35]State of New York, 1979–1980 Regular Sessions, 7103-D, Article 28, para. 880.

[36]Adopted by the Board of Directors of the American Occupational Medical Association (23 July 1976), as reprinted in *Bulletin of the New York Academy of Medicine* 54 (September 1978), Appendix: 818–19.

[37]OSHA regulations, Section III g, p. 35280.

have no affirmative duty to provide the *content* of these records; only their *existence* must be disclosed. A direct employee request is necessary for disclosure of content.

The implications of worker ignorance about certain health hazards in many industries received compelling expression in testimony before an OSHA hearing by a worker exposed to the toxic agent dibromochloropropane (DBCP), an agent present in many work environments where occupational physicians are employed: "We had no warning that DBCP exposure might cause sterility, testicular atrophy, and perhaps cancer. If we had known that these fumes could possibly cause the damage that we have found out it probably does cause, we would have worn equipment to protect ourselves. As it was, we didn't have enough knowledge to give us the proper respect for DBCP. Had we been warned of these dangers, some may not have accepted employment in the first place."[38]

Physicians like Dr. Young may be the only source of the knowledge that a request for information should be made by the worker, and such disclosures to workers clearly could conflict with the employer's interest. As Elihu Richter points out,[39] the difficulty with such access rights is that unless workers *request* the information, they may not possess even minimal risk information. If the right to know in the workplace is to be adequately protected, many contexts suggest that there must be an affirmative duty to disclose information about health hazards to workers in addition to a duty to honor worker-initiated requests for access to records. This is a serious problem for occupational physicians.

The case of Dr. Young provides an example. Because the company has undertaken efforts to reduce the levels of cotton dust, employees may believe they no longer face significant risk. They simply may not know that significant health hazards remain. In addition, since the disorders and diseases caused by cotton dust take months or even years to develop, employees may not know that they are now at risk until it is too late. Employees in these mills thus may lack the base-line information that would lead them to request the detailed information about health hazards that Dr. Young possesses. If the employee's right is to be meaningful, the needed information should be disclosed. Moreover, the beneficence model requires that the physician act to reduce unnecessary health risks to the employees. The autonomy and beneficence models therefore converge on a strong obligation of disclosure.

Employers often discourage the dissemination of information about hazards for understandable economic reasons. These include not only considerations of profitability but also the impact on productivity caused by the

---

[38]OSHA regulations, p. 35222.

[39]Elihu D. Richter, "The Worker's Right to Know: Obstacles, Ambiguities, and Loopholes," 341.

tension and strain resulting from disclosure. Moreover, occupational physicians have observed that a not insignificant fraction of the workforce begins to claim headaches, sick leave, and the like—and some even mimic the described symptoms of the disease—merely by virtue of the suggestion that they may be susceptible to it. Occupational physicians with obligations to employers must therefore think through disclosures such as those suggested by Dr. Young with great care. They cannot escape balancing the conflicting interests of different parties in this context.

Informed Consent and the Right to Know. One way to resolve this conflict is to appeal to developed models of disclosure obligations and the right to know, as presently found in literature on informed consent and informed refusal.[40] Unfortunately, neither this literature nor our conclusions in chapter three transfer easily to the situation of the occupational physician. Informed consent standards were fashioned for contexts involving fiduciary relationships between physicians and patients, where there are recognized moral and legal obligations to disclose known risks and benefits associated with a proposed treatment. No parallel obligation traditionally has been *legally* recognized in nonfiduciary relationships, such as that between management and workers and that between employer-provided physicians and workers. There is no reasonable analogy drawn in contemporary law, moral philosophy, or medical ethics between a traditional fiduciary relationship and the employer-employee relationship or the occupational physician-employee relationship. Nor can any direct analogy be made to union-employee relationships, for unions, too, are not fiduciaries in the eyes of the law. Indeed, workers often do not want information about their health transmitted to unions. Consequently neither employers nor unions have a fiduciary obligation in law to warn actively of risks or to disclose data discovered during examinations. Employers can be sued for fraudulent misrepresentation of the risks of a job, but not for failure to disclose risk. Following this line of reasoning, the occupational physician may justifiably take his or her overriding obligations to be to the employer.

Our analysis of conflicts of obligation caused for the occupational physician by the third-party interests of employers shows the same pattern of justification that we identified in the previous sections, but with an added complexity introduced by the peculiar nature of employers' interests. Some conflicts for the occupational physician arise because the employee is properly regarded as a patient whose health interests are in conflict with the economic interests of the employer. Under both the beneficence and au-

---

[40]The issue of the employees' right to know could also be profitably explored through an examination of the literature on the analogous issue of the patients' right to know, and in particular, the literature on patient access to medical records. For a discussion of the relationship between this literature and the issue of workers' rights of access to employer records, see the OSHA regulations, pp. 35228–36.

tonomy models, disclosure is generally obligatory, even if such a course of action is not in the employer's interest. Nevertheless, moral dilemmas emerge if the occupational physician is also an employee or is under contract, with obligations to an employer similar to those of other employees. The occupational physician faces a conflict of sometimes equally compelling obligations to employee-patient and employer. Like his or her colleagues in research, in HMOs, and in contact with parents, the occupational physician is squeezed between the interests of patients and those of third parties. Moreover, there are situations in which the interests of the employer justifiably override the interests of the patient or employee. In addressing these conflicts, the physician is perhaps best advised to rely predominantly on the virtue of honesty: Both employer and employee should be apprised of how the physician weighs their competing interests. This approach enhances trust and creates more stable expectations on the part of both parties, while avoiding at least some confusion and unnecessary tension.

The Local Community and the State

Physicians have long accepted obligations to protect the health and welfare of the communities in which they reside. The first *Code of Ethics* of the American Medical Association, for example, contains a lengthy section on the obligations of physicians to "the public," including the care of those who are sick and poor, as well as general public health responsibilities.[41] This position had been defended in the previous century by Johann Peter Frank, a German physician who held high posts in government and academia. His view of the physician's obligations to the community stems from a strong general principle of beneficence directed toward public health: "Medical police [Frank's term for the public health role of physicians] . . . is an art of defense, a model of protection of people and their animal helpers against the deleterious consequences of dwelling together in large numbers, but especially of promoting their physical well-being so that people will succumb as late as possible to their eventual fate from the many physical illnesses to which they are subject."[42] In a more recent article in the *New England Journal of Medicine*, Dr. Fitzhugh Mullan similarly argues that primary care and community medicine should be united in what he terms "community-oriented primary care."[43] Under this proposal, the physician is obligated not only to care for his or her patients

[41]American Medical Association, "Code of Ethics," in *Proceedings of the National Medical Convention, 1846–1847*, reprinted in *Ethics in Medicine*, ed. Stanley Reiser et al. (Cambridge: MIT Press, 1977), pp. 33–34.

[42]Johann Peter Frank, *A System of Complete Medical Police*, trans. Erna Lesky (Baltimore: Johns Hopkins University Press, 1976), p. 12.

[43]Fitzhugh Mullan, "Community-Oriented Primary Care," *New England Journal of Medicine* 307 (21 October 1982): 1076–78.

but to attend to "the overall problems of the community," including activities to "promote health and prevent disease."[44]

Case Study: The Contraction of Syphilis. Obligations to the community can conflict with obligations generated by the two models of moral responsibility, as the following case illustrates. Dr. Ralph Walker has just informed his patient, William Johnson, that he has syphilis. Mr. Johnson admits to Dr. Walker that he almost certainly contracted the disease during the course of an extramarital affair. He asks Dr. Walker to say nothing to anyone about his condition, for fear of his wife's reaction. What are Dr. Walker's responsibilities in this situation?

It is in Mr. Johnson's best interests (under the beneficence model) for these other parties to know about his condition so that preventive measures can be taken to protect him, as well as them. It is not difficult to imagine, however, that even in the face of such information, Mr. Johnson may insist that his physician maintain confidentiality. Any unauthorized disclosure of information about Mr. Johnson to third parties, including his wife, is prima facie wrong because such disclosure violates the physician's obligation to maintain Mr. Johnson's confidentiality. At the same time, not disclosing the condition to Mrs. Johnson is prima facie wrong becaue she will not be protected from an undeserved threat to her health. The same is true of Mr. Johnson's extramarital partner. The physician is faced with a genuine dilemma: On the one hand, Dr. Walker has an obligation to protect third parties from unnecessary compromise of their present health status, thus reducing the threat to their best interests. On the other hand, maintenance of medical confidentiality is an equally significant obligation. It is not clear how this dilemma should be resolved.

Because syphilis is a reportable disease in every jurisdiction in the United States, Dr. Walker has a clearly justifiable legal obligation to disclose Mr. Johnson's condition to local public health authorities. Government is charged in U.S. law with protecting the public welfare, and control of communicable disease is one way of discharging this obligation. The state's obligations to promote the health interests of Mrs. Johnson and Mr. Johnson's extramarital partner derive from this fundamental source, and the physician's moral obligation to override Mr. Johnson's right to confidentiality in favor of these third parties increases as the threat to health increases. Any reasonable person would want to have such protection if ignorant of the circumstances; thus the obligation to disclose is also based in both beneficence and respect for the autonomy of the third parties.

Suppose that Mr. Johnson informs Dr. Walker that Mrs. Johnson is three months pregnant and that they continue to have intercourse. If Mr. Johnson should cause his wife to become infected—indeed, he may already have done so—and, should an infection go undetected—a distinct possibil-

---

[44]Ibid., 1077.

ity in the case of syphilis in women—their baby may become infected, with potentially serious results that include blindness and possible brain damage. In these circumstances, it seems obvious that the physician's primary moral obligation is not to maintain Mr. Johnson's confidentiality but to protect innocent third parties: the future infant, as well as Mrs. Johnson and Mr. Johnson's extramarital partner. The principle of beneficence in these circumstances overrides Mr. Johnson's autonomy rights (and overrides the directives of the autonomy model) because the problems Mr. Johnson will face when his wife discovers the extramarital affair can probably be ameliorated, but the handicaps the infant will suffer are serious and irreversible. The physician's obligation to protect the future infant again seems overriding because no other action properly balances the goods and harms at stake.

Furthermore, the obligations of the physician do not stop with the local community because medicine cannot escape the impact of legislation, case law, and public policy. We must therefore consider third-party interests of the state as well. Serious attention to the state's interests is a recent development in contemporary medical ethics. Daniel Callahan, for example, has argued that a medical ethics that focuses exclusively on the patient-physician relationship is radically incomplete, because it omits attention to health policy and to society's legitimate interests in the activities of physicians.[45] Others have suggested that medical ethics must make health policy its *primary* emphasis.[46] These issues range beyond the scope of this book, and our treatment of them must take a modest form. Our exclusive focus will be on conflicts generated for the physician, as illustrated in the case that follows.

Case Study: Providing Information in Third-Party Payment.   William Pierce is a fifty-five-year-old man who has had adult-onset diabetes for the past ten years. He has been maintained on insulin and a modified diet to control his condition. He has, however, not always been diligent in taking his insulin and he has had several episodes of complications, including a diabetic coma requiring hospitalization. In the past two years, Mr. Pierce has developed hypertension, which is also controlled with a pharmacological regimen. Finally, Mr. Pierce suffers from congestive heart failure and experiences shortness of breath upon mild exertion.

---

[45]Daniel Callahan, "Contemporary Biomedical Ethics," *New England Journal of Medicine* 302 (29 May 1980): 1228–33.

[46]See Roy Branson, "The Scope of Bioethics: Individual and Social," and Albert F. Jonsen and Andre Hellegers, "Conceptual Foundations for an Ethics of Medical Care," both in *Ethics and Health Policy,* ed. Robert M. Veatch and Roy Branson (Cambridge: Ballinger Publishing Co., 1976), pp. 5–16, 17–33. Others, e.g., Paul Ramsey, have demurred, arguing instead that medical ethics should retain a primary emphasis on the obligations of physicians to patients. See his "Conceptual Foundations for an Ethics of Medical Care: A Response," in *Ethics and Health Policy,* pp. 35–55.

Eighteen months ago Mr. Pierce lost his job as a press operator when the newspaper for which he worked went out of business. He has been unable to find work and his unemployment benefits have run out. At a regular office visit, Mr. Pierce tells his physician that he will not be able to pay for this or future visits. He has exhausted his savings. His wife is only a part-time employee, and so does not qualify for private health insurance through her employer. Her salary, though meager, disqualifies them for public health reimbursement programs. His three children, he says, are not able to help out because they have families of their own, and each has heavy financial responsibilities. Mr. Pierce tells his physician that, if he were certified as fully disabled, state programs would pay the full cost of his physician's bills, medication, and hospitalization. He then requests that his physician complete a form he has brought along, in the hope that the state agency will declare him one hundred percent disabled.

The choices open to Mr. Pierce's physician are the following. On the one hand, his physician could describe Mr. Pierce's medical problems by placing a strong, somewhat exaggerated—but not untrue—emphasis on the stress that work might cause to Mr. Pierce's cardiovascular system. The result might well be that Mr. Pierce would be declared disabled by the state after receiving the physician's report. Mr. Pierce would then have the financial means to continue to see his physician for his regular visits, pay for his medication, and not suffer from anxiety over the financial disaster of hospitalization. This response would presumably be acting in Mr. Pierce's best interests because it fulfills the obligations of both the autonomy model, in response to his request, and the beneficence model, in avoiding for Mr. Pierce the unnecessary harms of medical complications that might ensue should he not receive adequate care and supervision.

Alternatively, Mr. Pierce's physician could simply state that the patient has adult-onset diabetes, hypertension, and congestive heart failure. State authorities would then make their own decision about whether to declare Mr. Pierce disabled. It is likely in these circumstances that they would not declare disability because many jobs do not require physical exertion. As a consequence, Mr. Pierce may then be unable to pay for hospitalization, his physician visits, and the medication that he needs to control his medical problems. That is, the physican could fulfill his or her responsibilities to the state, but perhaps at the price of not fulfilling obligations to Mr. Pierce based on the two models of moral responsibility.

A final alternative is that Mr. Pierce's physician could offer to accept him as a patient at a minimal or even no fee. However, Mr. Pierce would still face the costs of medication and possible hospitalization. The first course of action clearly places the patient's best medical interests above the competing interests of the state. The second alternative makes protecting the interests of the state the overriding consideration. Offering to continue taking care of Mr. Pierce at reduced cost is something of a middle ground between the two. It is clearly supererogatory (that is, above and beyond duty) and based on the ideal of placing the patient's interests first.

These conflicting alternatives are created for the physician by a public policy designed to limit eligibility for full reimbursement of health care costs by the state. Such policies allocate different levels of health care services to different sectors of the population. As such, they deal with patients in the aggregate, not as individuals. The physician finds patients lodged in a system designed for aggregates and must calculate how best to treat them as individuals. In this respect the third-party interests of the state are indeed remote from those of the patient.

However, although the interests of the state and of public policy can be remote from the individual patient's best interest, this is not alone a sufficient reason to dismiss them as morally irrelevant. Such public policies might be justified in terms of justice or utility. This prompts the question, How should the physician take account of fair allocation policies when they require actions contrary to the best interests of patients?

The Weight of Principles of Social Justice.   Asking this question renders the conflict faced by Mr. Pierce's physician more acute. To act in Mr. Pierce's best interests is not simply to override the interests of the state. It is also to claim, implicitly and without argument, that, as Hans Jonas puts it, "the physician is obligated to the patient *and to no one else.*"[47] This version of the principle, "The best interests of my patient come first," now takes on a new dimension: It paradoxically justifies the physician in committing the resources of society to the care of his or her patient when society, under legitimate requirements of justice, let us assume, may have no obligation to provide the resources. This approach allows the patient's best interests to override considerations of social justice.

By contrast, to assume that the physician always should follow the demands of social justice raises its own set of problems. In making decisions about patients in the aggregate, public policy tends to ignore the patient whose medical needs are far greater than a level of need averaged over all the individuals in the aggregate. That is, a just health care policy may be adequate to meet the basic needs of most individuals in the aggregate, without being adequate to meet the basic needs of those in that aggregate who might be among the worst off or the most vulnerable, as Mr. Pierce arguably is. In such circumstances, "The interests of my patient come first" becomes an ideal to be satisfied wherever possible, but not an absolute guide to the resolution of conflict. The theoretical reason is that principles of justice, like those of respect for autonomy and beneficence, are prima facie principles that can be overriding in determining the physician's obligations.

[47]Hans Jonas, "Philosophical Reflections on Experimenting with Human Subjects," in his *Philosophical Essays: From Ancient Creed to Technological Man* (Englewood Cliffs, N.J.: Prentice-Hall, Inc., 1974), pp. 1–31. (Emphasis added.)

Although our analysis in general has minimized the weight of the state's interests, it deserves at least passing notice that in some cultures and political units, the roles of the state and the legitimacy of appeals to social justice have been far more pronounced. The "Oath of a Doctor in the Soviet Union" is an official oath made compulsory in 1971. It specifies "the moral responsibility and the duty of a doctor to Soviet Society." The last and most important of the five items in the oath is the following: "I solemnly swear . . . to preserve and develop the noble traditions of our country's medicine; in all my actions to be guided by the principles of communist morality; to remember always a Soviet doctor's lofty calling and responsibility to the people and the Soviet State." In Soviet health policy it is clear, as Michael Ryan puts it, that "when faced with a choice between acting in the interests of his patient and the interests of the State, a doctor, is, so to speak, 'honor bound' to resolve this dilemma in favour of the State."[48]

Many other writers and states have held that when health policies are demonstrably consistent with the requirements of justice, they may create obligations that properly override obligations based in the principle, "My patient comes first." Such a conclusion is not without long historical precedent, as we saw when we considered Johann Peter Frank's notion of "medical police." Frank's concept was that the primary obligations of the physician are owed not merely to the local community, but to the *state*, and in particular to the monarch. Obligations to the individual patient are therefore secondary. Frank argues that physicians have compelling public health responsibilities, a major concern at that time with the emergence and enlargement of modern cities accompanied by problems of housing, clean air, and sanitation.[49]

Frank's approach and that of the Soviet government are regarded by many contemporary physicians as radically different from their understandings of their obligations to patients. This is no surprise, given the emphasis on the patient's best interests and the two models of moral responsibility that we examined in the earlier chapters of this book. There is, however, an additional reason. In Western democracies there is a deep-seated political reluctance to create a *primary* obligation on the part of professionals (and indeed on the part of citizens generally) to the central government or state. It is thus for reasons of political philosophy, as well as for its deep conflict with the two models of professional responsibility, that the notion of a primary obligation to the state appears as jarring as it does.

Nonetheless, even in Western nations, conflicts emanating from health policy exhibit the same three-part pattern of justification that we have seen

[48]Michael Ryan, "USSR Letter: Aspects of Ethics (1)," *British Medical Journal* 6190, vol. 2 (8 September 1979): 585–86. All the quotations in this paragraph are taken from this source. Other cultural perspectives on the responsibilities of physicians are discussed by Robert Veatch in his *A Theory of Medical Ethics* (New York: Basic Books, 1982), Chapter 3.

[49]Johann Peter Frank, *A System of Complete Medical Police*, passim.

to characterize conflicts involving parents, health care institutions, educational and research institutions, and employers. In each case, ethics can offer no compelling argument for the conclusion that the interests of one party *always* override the interests of another. Regrettably, discussion on these matters in the literature of medical ethics has only recently been undertaken, and is still in its early stages.[50]

CONCLUSION

We conclude that the principle, "The best interests of my patient come first" is not absolute. It is a rebuttable presumption that must sometimes give way to the principle, "The interests of third parties come first." Although there is no well-developed *model* of moral responsibility to third parties, any adequate account of the physician's moral responsibilities must accommodate interests of parties such as the family, health care institutions, medical education and research, future generations of patients, employers, the local community, and the state. For each, a range of conflicts is present for the physician. Some forms of conflict are best resolved in favor of the patient, others present genuine dilemmas, and still others are best resolved in favor of the third party.

The prima facie nature of moral principles of duty has been a constant theme in this book. In a world where only one moral principle, one model of moral responsibility, and one theory of third-party interests reigned supreme, physicians might be able to avoid the conflicts we have examined. If our analysis is correct, however, this is a misleading expectation for medical ethics, as for ethics generally. Hence, we have frequently argued that physicians must rely heavily on virtues such as respectfulness, honesty, tact, discretion, compassion, sympathy, and tolerance. The importance of this reliance must not be understated. These virtues enliven and nourish the humanity of medicine, sometimes transforming difficult problems of conflict into dignified and humane interchanges.

[50]See Robert M. Veatch and Roy Branson, eds., *Ethics and Health Policy;* Earl Shelp, ed., *Justice and Health Care* (Dordrecht, Holland: D. Reidel Publishing Co., 1981); *Journal of Medicine and Philosophy* 4 (1979), entitled "Rights to Health Care."

Index